DEPARTMENT OF HEALTH AND SOCIAL SECURITY

Sharing Resources for Health in England

Report of the Resource Allocation Working Party

London: Her Majesty's Stationery Office

ISBN 0 11 320227 X

Contents

Preface

The Resource Allocation Working Party was appointed in May 1975 with the following terms of reference:

> 'To review the arrangements for distributing NHS capital and revenue to RHAs, AHAs and Districts respectively with a view to establishing a method of securing, as soon as practicable, a pattern of distribution responsive objectively, equitably and efficiently to relative need and to make recommendations.'

Details of membership and the methods of working adopted by the Working Party are recorded in Annex A.

The First Interim Report of the Working Party was delivered in August 1975. Annex B records the responses to the recommendations in that Report and the action taken upon them.

In this Report, we present our conclusions based upon over a year's study of the many and complex issues associated with the problem of establishing a method of securing a pattern of distribution of the resources available to the NHS in England in a way that is responsive to the relative needs of the populations which it serves.

In presenting this Report we wish to acknowledge with gratitude the very considerable help given by those who joined our Working Groups and by the many officers and professionals in the Department and the NHS who responded readily and uncomplainingly to our not infrequent requests for information, advice and guidance. Without their invaluable contributions our task might well have proved impossible to discharge. We take the opportunity also to express our very special appreciation of the exemplary efficiency with which we have been supported at all times by our Secretariat.

September 1976

CHAPTER I

Resource Allocation – The Nature of the Problem – Definitions and Distinctions

INTRODUCTION AND BACKGROUND

1.1 There is ample evidence to demonstrate that demand for health care throughout the world is rising inexorably. England has no immunity from this phenomenon. And because it can also be shown that supply of health care actually fuels further demand, it is inevitable that the supply of health care services can never keep pace with the rising demands placed upon them. Demand will always be one jump ahead. This is a problem for Government and society in general and not, fortunately, one to which the Working Party was called upon to address its mind. We mention it at the beginning of this Report, however, to emphasize two points. Firstly that the resources available to the NHS are bound to fall short of requirements as measured by demand criteria and secondly that supply of facilities has an important influence on demand in the locality in which they are provided.

1.2 Supply of health facilities is, in England as elsewhere, also variable and very much influenced by history. The methods used to distribute financial resources to the NHS have, since its inception, tended to reflect the inertia built into the system by history. They have tended to increment the historic basis for the supply of real resources (eg facilities and manpower); and, by responding comparatively slowly and marginally to changes in demography and morbidity, have also tended to perpetuate the historic situation.

1.3 This led us in our Interim Report to interpret the underlying objective of our terms of reference as being to secure, through resource allocation, that there would eventually be equal opportunity of access to health care for people at equal risk. We reaffirm this view. It has involved us in seeking criteria which are broadly responsive to relative need, not supply or demand, and to employ those criteria to establish and quantify in a relative way the differentials of need between different geographical locations. For practical purposes these geographic locations must correspond with those into which the NHS is organized to administer the delivery of health care, viz, Regions, Areas and Districts.

1.4 In searching for criteria which are responsive in this way, we have had perforce to consider only those criteria, the supporting statistical data for which are readily available and reliable at all three levels of disaggregation required. We have further taken as an aim the desirability of keeping the methods proposed as simple as possible, consistent with the overall objective. The degree of refinement necessary is to some extent a matter of judgment, but we have not by any means regarded perfection in this context as an aim. On the contrary, we have rejected many approaches which might have made the criteria more sensitive, but which on examination would have led to much greater complexity with little significant change in the result.

1.5 *Resource allocation is concerned with the distribution of financial resources which are used for the provision of real resources. In this sense it is concerned with the means rather than the end. We have not regarded our remit as being concerned with how the resources are deployed.* This must be a matter for the administering Authorities and is essentially part of their policy-making, planning and decision-making functions in response to central guidelines on national policies and priorities. Resource allocation will clearly have an important influence on the discharge of those functions and be the most critical guideline within which they have to be discharged. This serves, however, to emphasize the importance, as our terms of reference direct, of ensuring that the availability of the finite resource at the NHS's disposal should be determined in relation to criteria of need.

CRITERIA OF NEED

Size of Population
1.6 Health care is for people and clearly the primary determinant of need must be the size of the population. This must therefore be the basic divisor used to distribute the resource available to each level required.

Population Make-up
1.7 The make-up of the population is, however, critical. People do not have identical needs for health care. For example, the elderly (men and women aged 65 and over) form about 14% of the total population, yet they

occupy more than half the non-psychiatric hospital beds (excluding maternity). Women have needs different from men, and children too are heavy users of health care facilities. Similarly, patterns of morbidity are different between the sexes at different ages. Thus the age/sex make-up of the population needs to be taken into account as well as its size.

Morbidity

1.8 Even when differences due to age and sex are fully accounted for, populations of the same size and make-up display different morbidity characteristics. The reasons are simple enough to guess but harder to quantify; environment, social circumstances, heredity, occupation etc all play a part. But a population-based measure of need which takes no account of different patterns of morbidity would ignore geographic variations which, on the data available, are significant.

Cost

1.9 The costs of providing care in response to need are also variable. Some conditions are very expensive to treat, others less so. It is not enough to use criteria which predict the likely incidence of the more expensive forms of care, unless at the same time some account is taken of the differential cost involved. Furthermore, the costs of exactly the same form of care may vary from place to place depending on local variations in market forces. A clear example of this is the weighting paid to staff employed in the London area.

Health Care Across Administrative Boundaries

1.10 The populations for which the administering Authorities are responsible for delivering health care are primarily those who reside within their geographic boundaries. In some cases these responsibilities are adjusted to take account of people residing in overlap areas – by means of formal agency or extra-territorial management arrangements. For resource allocation purposes the population needs to be that for which the Authority exercises a management responsibility.

1.11 But these arrangements do not take account of patients who receive care outside the managed area of their particular Authority. Patient flows across boundaries result from the fact that few Areas and Districts are entirely self-sufficient in terms of the services they provide. In some cases these 'deficiencies' are planned, eg Regional specialties, in others they are unplanned and are often the inevitable consequence of new and arbitrary administrative boundaries not matching established patterns of health care delivery. To a large extent unplanned patient flows are also a measure of geographical disparity in health care provision. Whether patient flows are from choice or necessity, the populations used for revenue allocations need to be adjusted to take account of the movement. And such adjustment ought also to reflect the different costs of care involved.

Medical and Dental Education

1.12 The NHS has a responsibility to provide clinical facilities for the teaching of students qualifying through the University Medical Schools. Service facilities which are used for medical and dental education are more costly to provide. The incidence of these costs is, however, unrelated either to the size or to the needs of the populations served by the hospitals where medical and dental education is undertaken. Means must therefore be found of identifying the additional costs necessarily involved and protecting those costs from the effects of allocation processes based upon population and service need criteria.

Capital Investment

1.13 Health services require considerable capital investment in buildings, plant and equipment. Whilst the need for capital investment may to a considerable extent be measurable by criteria similar to those used for determining need for current expenditure, there is one significant difference. As mentioned earlier in this chapter, the distribution of capital stock is still very much influenced by the historic patterns of health care delivery. There are not only geographic inequalities in the quantity of stock available but also in its age and condition. Nor do these factors of quantity and quality go hand in hand. Regions which are well provided in quantitative terms may, for the same historic reasons, have a large proportion of ageing stock. Furthermore, the effects of population movement, demographic change and the redefinition of administrative boundaries have all exacerbated the 'mislocation' problem.

1.14 Hitherto these factors have not been directly recognised in the arrangements for allocating capital resources. Although it poses difficult problems in assessment, we believe that they cannot continue to be ignored. Indeed we regard the relationship between capital and current expenditure to be crucial to the balanced development of health services. Obvious though this statement may appear, there seems to us to be ample evidence to support the view that capital expenditure has either been permitted to dominate and sometimes distort patterns of development or, to put it another way, its important characteristic as an investment for the future has been sacrificed in the interests of preserving consumption at a particular level.

INFORMATION PROBLEMS

1.15 Criteria of the kind mentioned above can be used to establish geographic differences in the need for health care and thus to provide a basis for resource allocation. The reliability and acceptability of the recommendations made later in our Report are to a large extent dependent, as we have said, on the information available. One of our main stumbling blocks has been the lack of relevant information in a suitable form. Broad demographic information is available from population censuses – though inter-censal change presents some problems – while more detailed demographic and social information can be obtained from the General Household Survey, though there are limits on the uses which can be made of it. Information on hospital service utilisation is available from the data processed for Hospital Activity Analysis (HAA), the Hospital Inpatient Enquiry (HIPE), the Mental Health Enquiry (MHE) and other periodic censuses. Data on community care are much more difficult to come by and information about the costs of health care and the way in which they break down between different specialties and functions is somewhat limited. Survey information on hospital stock is limited to age and size, and takes no account of facilities or condition, other than an indication of maintenance backlog; information on other health buildings is even more restricted. We are conscious of the probability that any allocation method based upon the data available may be open to challenge on grounds which will be difficult either to substantiate or refute. Had better data been available we would have used them. In spite of these reservations, however, we are convinced that the data we have used are sufficiently reliable to support the conclusions and methods we propose. That they might be refined we accept, but at the cost in time and money of considerable further research – an issue to which we turn later in this Report.

1.16 Not enough is known about the determinants of health needs. Even where particular factors can be seen to play a part in causing health need, it is often difficult to quantify the relationship and draw upon reliable information about when and where they occur. Health programmes are not the only means of improving health in a locality. We recognise the important influences of other factors, eg housing, environmental health facilities, working conditions etc. Except in the sense that they all have an impact on the morbidity of populations, we cannot take them into account. They are the province of other social programmes and the extent to which they react with the health care programme is not an issue with which we are equipped to deal. We welcome the initiatives being taken, however,

11

through the Joint Approach to Social Policy and the Review of Social Services and we hope that our work will make a contribution to their consideration of much wider problems.

THE PHASING OF CHANGE

1.17 Measuring relative need, complicated and difficult though it is, is only the beginning. This Report confirms the existence of large disparities between the way in which resources have traditionally been allocated to different parts of the country, and the way in which they would be allocated on our recommended criteria of relative need. Disparities of the order demonstrated could not be redressed at a stroke. Major facilities for health care such as hospitals take many years to build and the commissioning of these facilities and consequential re-use of existing buildings must also take into account manpower constraints and considerations of good personnel management. Time is therefore needed to plan, both for growth and for restraint, if changes are to take place in a way which best serves the interests of the community while safeguarding those of the staff in the NHS.

1.18 This is true in health service terms alone; it is reinforced when considering the effects of other services, such as those mentioned in paragraph 1.16 above, which interact with health provision. While it would be wrong to allow deficiencies in such services to be built into the assessment of a Health Authority's relative need for funds thus introducing or retaining permanent distortions in the local pattern of health services, we have to recognise that such deficiencies impose an added burden in certain places which cannot be ignored in the short term. These must therefore also be among the practical issues to be considered in determining the speed at which the disparities in health resources can be redressed.

THE SHAPE OF THIS REPORT

1.19 It has been necessary for us therefore to consider at each stage in our Report not only what changes are desirable but how rapidly they can take place. In the ensuing chapters we discuss, first in relation to RHAs and then in relation to AHAs and Districts, the measurement of relative need for revenue generally, for revenue in support of teaching and for capital; we consider in each case the constraints on change from year to year and, in our last chapter, we offer a synoptic view of the recommendations, comment on the balance between capital and revenue, and set out a plan for research and review to provide foundations for future improvements.

CHAPTER II Distribution of Revenue to Regional Health Authorities

SCOPE OF THIS CHAPTER

2.1 This chapter is concerned with revenue provision for health services provided by Health Authorities, whether delivered in teaching or non-teaching hospitals or in the community. Additional revenue costs arising from the presence of medical schools are dealt with in a separate chapter. We remain of the view first expressed in our Interim Report, that formulae should be the chief determinants of allocations from the DHSS to RHAs. We recognise that limited use of central reserves may be unavoidable: this is acceptable so long as it is kept to a minimum. Application of a formula to the distribution of all but this fraction of the revenue available for services entails three distinct logical steps:

2.1.1 The application of measures of relative need, to establish the share of available revenue to which each RHA would be entitled on the basis of need criteria alone. This share constitutes each RHA's 'revenue target', towards which it should be moving as fast as circumstances permit.

2.1.2 Establishing where each Authority stands now in relation to its revenue target. For RHAs, this means simply comparing the allocation actually received last year with the target allocation.

2.1.3 Determining how fast it is possible for each Authority to move from its present position towards its revenue target, bearing in mind practical constraints on the pace of change in whatever direction may be desirable.

SETTING REVENUE TARGETS FOR RHAs

The Population Base

2.2 As stated in Chapter I, the first criterion of relative need must be population. **For revenue purposes, we recommend that this should be the** estimate of the mid-year population of each Region nearest to the year for which allocations are made. In practice, for each allocation year this would probably be the mid-year estimate for the year two years earlier. At the time when allocations are made, this base is more up-to-date than that used for projections to the allocation year and is therefore preferable.

2.3 The base population will then require adjusting to take account of population characteristics and other factors which affect people's need for health care. Because need for different services manifests itself in diverse ways, we have found it necessary to weight population separately in respect of seven different aspects of health services, which are discussed one by one below. These separate weighted populations are then combined to give a single adjusted population reflecting the overall needs of the locality concerned. It must be stressed that the purpose of the analysis is wholly and solely to arrive at this final figure. It should *not* be taken as an indication of, or even as a guideline to the level of funding appropriate to the service categories. It has no relevance in this context. Allocation of resources to particular services is entirely a matter for local planning and decision in accordance with national and Regional guidelines. The way in which Authorities choose to exercise this freedom will, however, in due course, influence the national figures on which the analysis is based.

Measuring Need for Non-psychiatric In-patient Services
2.4 *Age and sex.* There is ample evidence to demonstrate that men, women, boys and girls of different ages place different demands on hospital in-patient services. The age/sex make-up of the population of different Regions has a significant effect upon the need of each population for resources. To reflect this, it is necessary to weight the population by the demands made by each age/sex group on services. The best available measure is the national utilisation of hospital beds. **We recommend, therefore, that the population of each Region be weighted to reflect the difference in age/sex composition by reference to the national pattern of non-psychiatric hospital bed utilisation.**

2.5 *Morbidity.* Need for hospital in-patient services is not, of course, a function of age and sex alone. Many other factors are known to play a part – social, occupational, hereditary, environmental etc. The difficulty is not in determining which factors are likely to be influential, but in quantifying their influence and in eliminating overlap between them. Figures are available, for example, on relative population densities and on social class structures, but we have not found it possible to relate this information

14

quantitatively to the need for health care. Furthermore, factors such as occupation, poverty, social class and pollution are likely to interact in ways which are not fully understood.

2.6 But it would not be necessary to take account of causal factors such as those mentioned above if it were possible to measure health care need directly. In our Interim Report we relied upon Regional in-patient and out-patient caseloads as an indicator of relative need over and above that arising from the age/sex structure of the population. We recognised that this had serious imperfections. Whilst numbers of cases clearly reflect need, they do so in terms of the available supply of services. Caseloads fail both to distinguish between degrees of need and to assess the extent to which need is unmet through lack of facilities. Waiting lists as one indicator of unmet need are also known to have questionable reliability. Moreover there is ample evidence to support the view that the level of supply has a significant influence on the level of demand. Need must, therefore, be measured by an indicator that is far less dominated by supply.

2.7 Statistics relating to payment of sickness benefit are more independent in this sense but do not apply to the whole of the population, important categories such as the elderly, children and many married women being excluded. There are also problems relating to the causes of incapacity as certified, and Regional differences may be partly attributable to industrial structure: the ability to continue to work despite the presence of morbid conditions may for example be influenced by the nature of employment. Moreover sickness absence does not necessarily imply a need for health care over and above that which can be provided by a GP. The General Household Survey provides evidence of differences in GP consultation rates and the prevalence of self-reported sickness between different parts of the country but the nature of the sampling frame does not permit compilation of statistics in terms of NHS boundaries. Self-reported sickness is not a direct measure of the need for health care resources and differences in the levels of reported sickness may be due in part to differences in the perception and reporting of sickness. Nor would the data on diagnostic category be sufficiently reliable for our purposes. Past ad hoc surveys of morbidity in various fields cannot usually be extrapolated to national level. The samples are usually small, the data rapidly become out of date and repetition would be a difficult and costly business.

2.8 The search for a reliable indicator, as independent as possible of supply, which could be used to assess Regional differences in need led us to examine the possibility of using mortality statistics as a proxy indicator of morbidity. Mortality statistics cover the whole population, are readily available and permit compilation by place of usual residence. The quality of the statistics, including analyses by cause of death, is high. The crude death rate shows a considerable Regional variation (maximum exceeds minimum by 38% for both males and females). Even when allowance is made for age structure – which has a marked effect on comparative death rates – the residual variation is still as high as 28% for males and 21% for females. Figure II–1 illustrates the variations. The reasons for the pattern of differential Regional mortality are not wholly understood but it is believed that Regional differences in morbidity explain the greater part of it and that statistics of relative differences in Regional morbidity, if they existed, would exhibit the same pattern as those for mortality.

2.9 Some support for this assumption is provided by a comparison of mortality rates, adjusted to take account of age and sex differences, with such Regional morbidity-related data as exist, similarly adjusted. The comparison reveals significant positive correlations. The maps in Figure II-2 show the broad similarity between Regional differences in mortality and in data derived from sickness benefit statistics and the General Household Survey. Problems in using this information directly in the allocation process have already been outlined but these are less critical in the context of establishing geographical correlations with mortality because these can be calculated for standard statistical regions.

2.10 Mortality statistics also present an opportunity to relate differential morbidity to health care need by reference to conditions in a way that no other sources permit. It is possible to examine the variation in mortality between Regions by diagnostic conditions – using the underlying not the associated causes of death – grouping the conditions according to the 17 chapter headings of the International Classification of Diseases (ICD). The statistic used is the Standardised Mortality Ratio (SMR) which compares the number of deaths actually occurring in a Region with those which would be expected if the national mortality ratios by age and sex were applicable to the population of that Region. In this way the unique pattern of mortality in each Region can be established, calculated separately for each condition or group of conditions.

2.11 Many of the commonest conditions – including some which lead to death – place relatively little demand on health care services. Others require expensive care, perhaps over a long period. This relationship can be estab-

16

Figure II-1 Charts illustrating effects for each RHB of standardising 1971 crude death rates for age

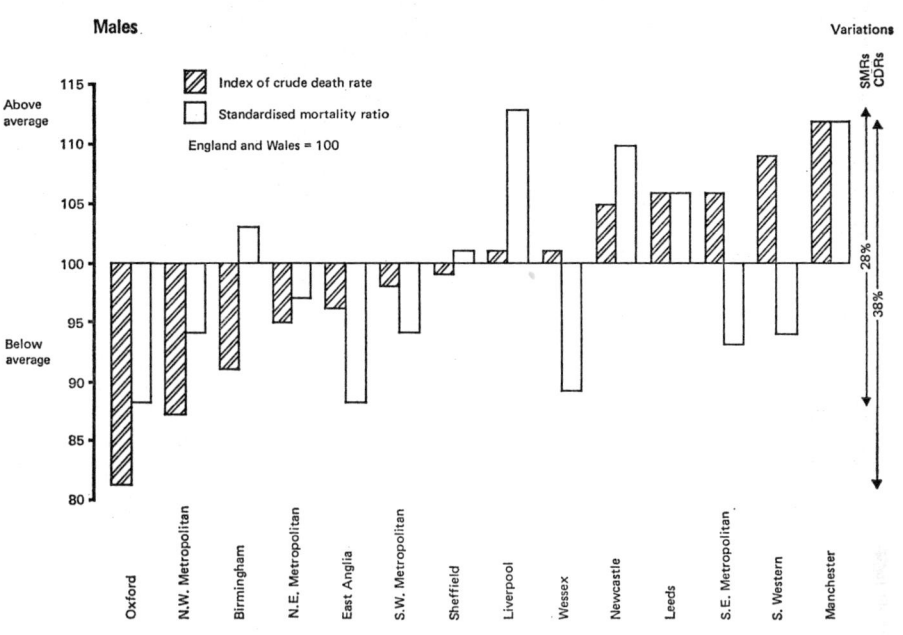

Males

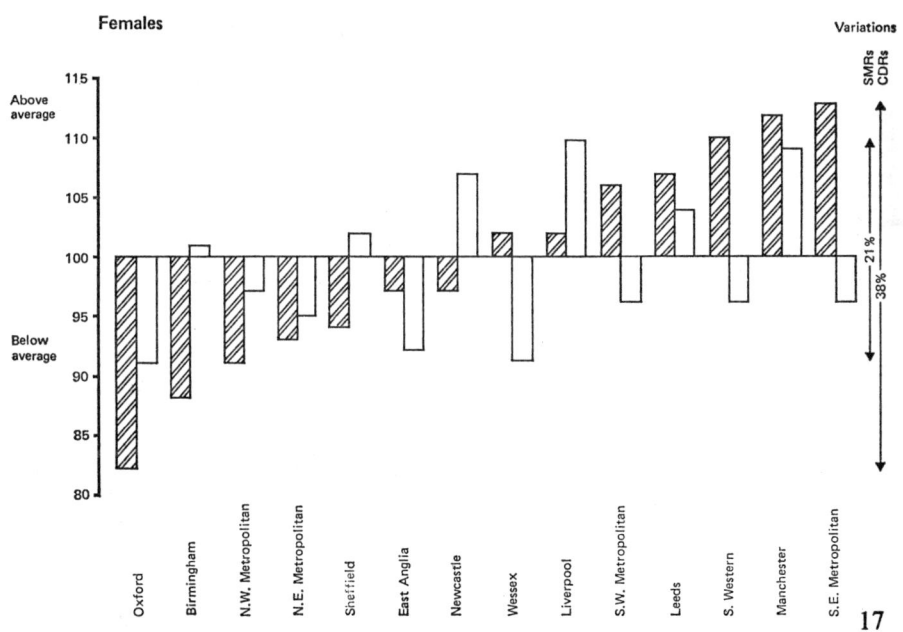

Females

17

18

Figure II-2 Standardised mortality ratios, 1972

Persons

Certified spells of incapacity standardised for age, 1972

Males*

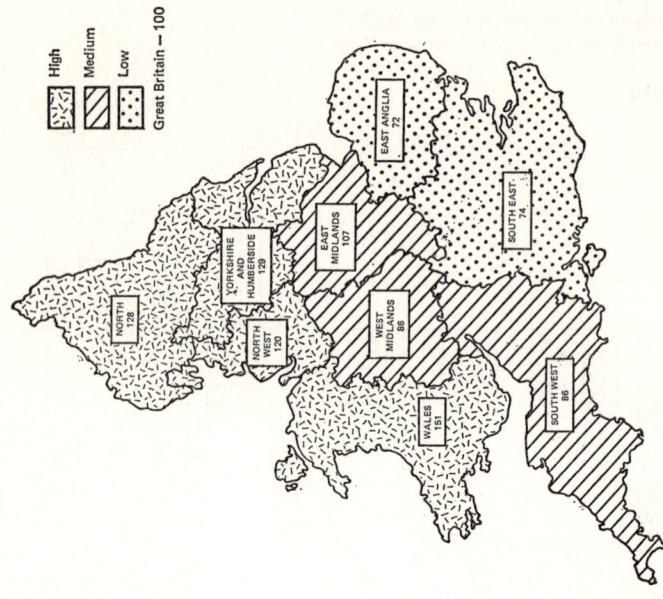

Standardised mortality ratios, 1972 (Persons):

High, Medium, Low — England and Wales — 100

NORTH 110
NORTH WEST 110
YORKSHIRE AND HUMBERSIDE 106
WALES 107
WEST MIDLANDS 103
EAST MIDLANDS 99
EAST ANGLIA 89
G.L.C. 97
OUTER MET 92
OUTER SOUTH EAST 88
SOUTH WEST 93

Certified spells of incapacity standardised for age, 1972 (Males*):

High, Medium, Low — Great Britain — 100

NORTH 128
NORTH WEST 120
YORKSHIRE AND HUMBERSIDE 129
WALES 151
WEST MIDLANDS 86
EAST MIDLANDS 107
EAST ANGLIA 72
SOUTH EAST 74
SOUTH WEST 86

Subdivisions of England and Wales are standard statistical regions

*Females have been excluded because of the large
proportion who are not insured for sickness benefit

Self reported chronic illness standardised
for age and sex, GHS 1972

Persons

High
Medium
Low
England and Wales — 100

Self reported acute illness standardised
for age and sex, GHS 1972

Persons

High
Medium
Low
England and Wales — 100

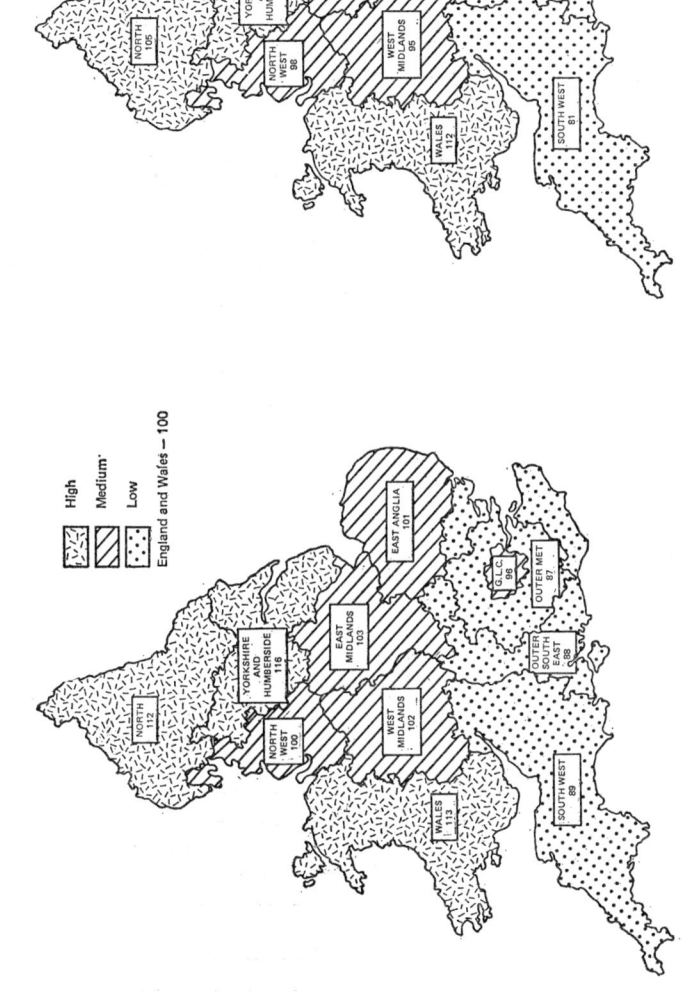

GHS data: Acute sickness is defined as restriction at any time during a two
week reference period of the level of normal activity caused by
illness or injury. Chronic sickness is defined as a state of long-
standing illness, disability or infirmity.

19

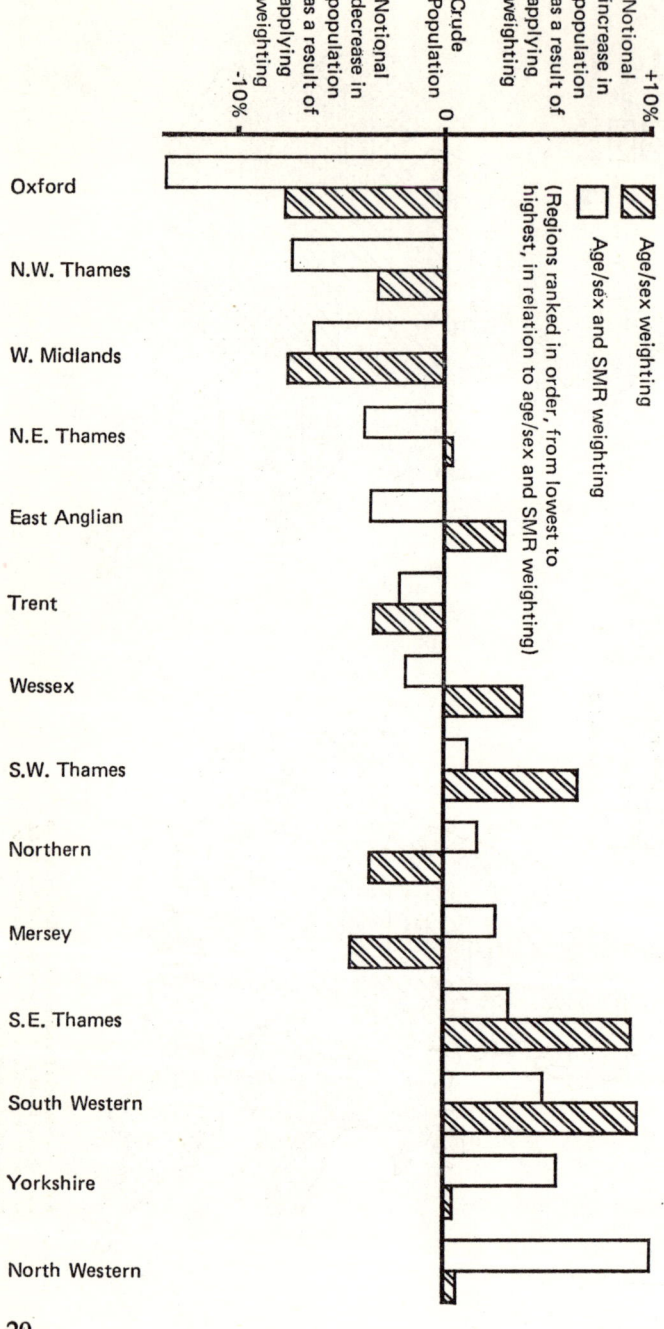

Figure II-3 Chart illustrating the effects of age/sex weighting and age/sex/SMR weighting (applied to each region's crude population)

(based on figures contained in Table C7)

lished by reference to the national figures of hospital bed utilisation for each condition category considered and incorporated in the calculation to provide the final link in the chain from mortality through morbidity to need for health services.

2.12 To each Region's population we have applied national age/sex utilisation rates for each individual group of conditions, calculated a standardised mortality ratio for each group and combined the two weighting factors for each condition. The effect of doing this is to produce a set of weighting factors independent of Regional differences in the supply of NHS facilities and reflecting morbidity differences between different parts of the country over and above those resulting from age and sex disparities. The method ensures that, in applying SMRs by condition, account is taken of the proportionate national bed utilisation for each condition. Figure II-3 shows how the results compare with those of a population weighting based on hospital utilisation analysed by age and sex alone.

2.13 As a result of the studies and analyses we have carried out, supported by the findings of research in related fields and expert advice, we have come to the conclusion that SMRs – adjusted in the way we propose – are the best available indicators of geographical variations in morbidity. And to ignore the considerable variations which this analysis displays would be to ignore a crucial factor in determining the relative needs for health care of different localities.

2.14 For certain conditions where mortality is very low – eg skin diseases and conditions of pregnancy – SMRs are unlikely to give a good guide to morbidity, and we have omitted these from our calculations. Age/sex weighting alone is a good indicator of the need for maternity services but it can be further improved by modifying the age/sex weighting for ICD Condition XI (conditions of pregnancy, childbirth, puerperium) to reflect fertility rates standardised for age, in the same way as other condition categories can be modified by SMRs.

2.15 There is evidence that other factors, eg marital status, are associated with the need for health care, but to add to those we have already proposed would strain the data to the point at which reliability was lost and incur a risk of double-counting. **We recommend that, in respect of acute non-psychiatric hospital in-patient services, the population weighted for age and sex by national bed utilisation for each condition should be adjusted to take into account condition-specific SMRs for each Region. SMRs for** conditions unlikely to lead to death, eg skin diseases, should not be used. For conditions of pregnancy, childbirth and puerperium, SMRs should be replaced by an index of fertility rates standardised for age.

2.16 *Cost-weighting.* The cost of providing health care differs according to the condition being treated. In principle, therefore, the weighting system described above ought to be improved by attaching differential costs to the utilisation data. In practice, this is one of the areas where information is weakest. It is not at present possible to establish costs relative to ICD conditions. We have, however, set in hand a study which may enable a broad distinction to be made between conditions requiring predominantly acute or non-acute care, and the results, which will not be available until the autumn, may make it possible to apply a form of cost-weighting pending the availability of better information.

2.17 *Movement of patients across administrative boundaries.* Allocations must reflect the populations served, not simply those who reside within the administrative boundary. Where a RHA is responsible for managing services located outside its own geographic Region under a formal agency arrangement, the population there should be credited to the managing Region and not the Region of residence. Similarly, the costs of care for people who cross Regional boundaries to receive hospital in-patient services or are treated in hospitals managed by other RHAs (ie extra-territorially managed hospitals) should be credited to the Region providing treatment, and debited to the Region in which they live. The adjustment should have regard to the average national cost of the kind of services provided, rather than to local costs which may be influenced by local policy decisions. **We therefore recommend that adjustments to weighted populations should be made to take account of inter-Regional patient flows costed on a national specialty basis.**

Measuring Need for Day- and Out-patient Services
2.18 All of the principles described in the foregoing paragraphs in relation to in-patient services apply, mutatis mutandis, to day- and out-patient services also. The necessary differences are:

2.18.1 *Age/sex weighting* should reflect national utilisation of services by out-patients and not that by in-patients, since the utilisation pattern is different between the two groups.

2.18.2 *Morbidity* among non-psychiatric day- and out-patients is just as likely to be reflected by SMRs as it is among in-patients. Unfortunately it is not practicable to break down utilisation of these services by ICD condition so as to apply a utilisation weighting similar to that recommended for non-psychiatric hospital in-patients. It is, however, possible to modify the age/sex weighting for these groups by applying the overall SMR for each Region. We have established that overall SMRs when applied to in-patients give broadly the same result as the condition-specific SMRs. Though less sensitive, overall SMRs may therefore be applied to non-psychiatric day- and out-patients.

2.18.3 *Movement of patients across administrative boundaries.* There are no statistics generally available to measure reliably the extent to which day- and out-patients cross Regional boundaries for services. We have searched for a different indicator which might be used as a proxy; but, after very full consideration, we have come to the conclusion that no assumptions as to the validity of any proxy can be made with any confidence. For example, whilst in-patient flows in some localities are thought to correspond approximately with out-patient flows, there is evidence to suggest that this correspondence is by no means general. We are not, therefore, in a position to make any recommendations save that we regard it as an urgent need to assemble better information about this group of patients, who represent a substantial and increasing proportion of NHS expenditure. Agency arrangements can and should be taken into account.

2.19 **We recommend that, in respect of non-psychiatric day- and out-patient services, the population of each Region should be weighted to reflect the national pattern of utilisation of these services by age and sex, adjusted in the case of non-psychiatric patients to take into account SMRs for each Region. The weighted population should be adjusted to take account of agency arrangements.**

Measuring Need for Community Services

2.20 The arguments and the data limitations applying to people using community services are similar to those for day- and out-patients. Age utilisation patterns nationally are different from those for other services and this should be taken into account. No sex analysis is possible. **We recommend that, in respect of community services, the population of each Region be weighted to reflect the national pattern of utilisation of these services by age, adjusted to take into account SMRs for each Region. The weighted population should be adjusted to take account of agency arrangements.**

Measuring Need for Ambulance Services

2.21 Examination of the available data on use of ambulance services, which, as for other community services, are far from comprehensive, reveals that by far the most significant explanation of Regional variation is crude population. Age/sex weightings cannot be applied on existing information. Demands on the services will, however, be affected by variations in morbidity, and the use of SMRs in the same way as for other community services is therefore desirable. The Working Party examined very carefully the possibility of taking variations in population density into account as well, but the study did not point conclusively to the need to adjust Regional allocations on this account. **We recommend that, in respect of ambulance services, the crude population of each Region be adjusted to take into account SMRs for each Region.**

Measuring Need for FPC Administration

2.22 FPC administration consumes a tiny proportion of the available revenue funds. There is no way of relating the need for this service to detailed indices of morbidity. **We therefore recommend that the index of need for FPC administration should be crude population.**

Measuring Need for Mental Illness Hospital In-patient Services

2.23 *Age and sex.* As for other services, there is evidence that the pattern of utilisation of mental illness services nationally differs between age/sex groups. **We recommend that the population of each Region be weighted to reflect the difference in age/sex composition by reference to the national pattern of mental illness hospital bed utilisation.**

2.24 *Morbidity.* Mortality is clearly not an appropriate measure for psychiatric morbidity, over and above that explained by age/sex variations, since mental illness is rarely the direct cause of death. We sought expert advice on the best indicators of need for these conditions in addition to age and sex. As in the case of physical illness, many potentially relevant indicators – social class, poverty, social isolation and others – would need considerable research before it was possible to include them in any formula. There is, however, quantitative evidence that non-married people place heavier demands on mental illness services nationally than do married people and the age/sex weighting can be modified to take account of this. **We recommend that, in respect of mental illness hospital in-patient services, marital status be used as an additional weighting factor to age and sex, pending the outcome of further research on other possible indicators.**

2.25 *Cost-weighting.* As for other services, the necessary information is lacking and must be added to the long list of research and data requirements.

2.26 *Movement of patients across administrative boundaries.* The same arguments apply as those adduced in paragraph 2.17 above in relation to non-psychiatric hospital in-patients and lead to similar conclusions, though it is not possible to include a cost-weighting because of the data deficiencies already mentioned. In addition, however, estimates of the need now likely to arise for mental illness services do not and cannot reflect the presence of long-stay patients, often admitted many years ago, whose original homes are in many cases no longer known. Such patients tend to be concentrated for historical reasons in relatively few places. **We recommend that patient flows should be taken into account in respect of mental illness hospital in-patient services with the modification that long-stay mentally ill patients admitted to hospital before the date of the last MHE Census should as a temporary measure be credited to the Region in which they are receiving care by means of an adjustment to reflect the actual as against the expected number of such patients based on weighted population. The adjustment should be phased out as existing imbalances are corrected, as the purpose is to recognise those imbalances due to historic crossing of boundaries not reflected in current patient flows.**

Measuring Need for Mental Handicap Hospital In-patient Services

2.27 Similar arguments apply to mental handicap services as to mental illness services, except that we have been unable to identify any criteria of need available for application in the short term other than age and sex differences. **We recommend that the population of each Region be weighted to reflect the national pattern of mental handicap hospital bed utilisation by people of different ages and each sex, and that the recommendations in paragraph 2.26 above should be applied in respect of mental handicap hospital in-patient services.**

Caseload

2.28 With the improvements outlined above, the retention of caseload as a separate element in the formula can no longer be justified. It is not a satisfactory indicator of need since the number of cases treated must depend to a large extent on the availability of facilities to treat them. It was retained for 1976/77 only as an expedient to make up for the inadequacies in the age/sex weighting of population. **We recommend that the caseload measure should now be abandoned.**

Figure II-4 The build-up of a revenue target

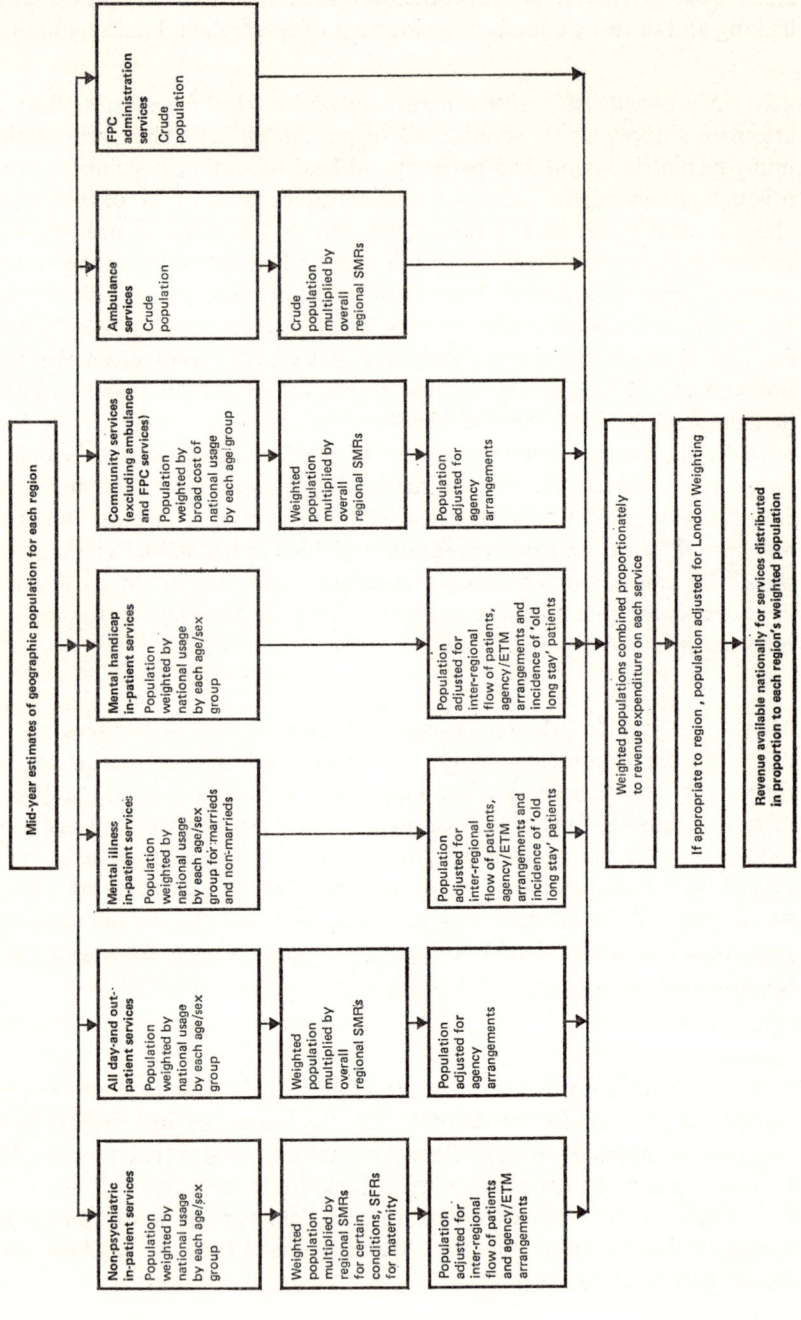

Establishing Revenue Target Allocations

2.29 Applying the recommendations in the preceding paragraphs produces seven separate weighted populations for each Region. **We recommend that these should be combined into a single weighted population for each Region in proportion to the most recent information available on relative expenditure nationally on the services concerned.** The revenue available for services nationally should then be notionally distributed in proportion to each Region's weighted population to arrive at the revenue target allocation for each RHA. The flow chart at Figure II-4 sets the whole process out in graphic form, while Annex C describes and illustrates in detail how the Working Party's recommendations could be put into practice and how the weighting factors are derived.

Differentials Caused by Market Variations

2.30 The proposals above assume implicitly that the unit costs of providing health care are the same in all Regions, or that any variations are so small that they can be safely ignored. There is evidence to suggest that market variations are significant and therefore that this assumption may not be valid.

2.31 NHS pay-scales are nationally negotiated and applied and this tends to level out unit manpower costs across the country as a whole. The fact that the NHS is virtually the sole employer of major professional groups, eg doctors, dentists, nurses and others, who therefore compete in a national rather than a local labour market, has a similar effect. On the other hand, the NHS is in competition with other employers for many groups of staff, particularly administrative and clerical and ancillary workers. Furthermore, even within a framework of national pay-scales some variation in labour costs can arise. Examples are distinction awards for medical staff, different amounts of overtime worked and discretion in grading particular posts and points of entry to salary scales. Where only poor-quality staff can be recruited, greater numbers may be needed. High turnover can also increase overheads, as can a need to resort to more use of part-time and agency staff. Difficulties in recruiting staff locally may lead to increased expenditure on providing transport and accommodation for recruits from further afield. To some extent, therefore, labour costs in the NHS are bound to vary in response to the general market forces operating in a particular locality.

2.32 Similarly, while central purchasing arrangements are likely to mitigate the effect of cost differentials for major supplies expenditure, certain goods and services are bought locally and will reflect local market conditions.

27

The cost of any services which have a high labour content and which are locally purchased will be affected by the market forces operating on employment generally in the locality concerned.

2.33 It is clear therefore that NHS costs can be affected by local market conditions. The questions to be answered are whether the variations can be quantified and if so whether they are likely to be significant. We have examined the information published in the New Earnings Survey for male and female manual and non-manual workers. The Survey is based on a 1% sample and is therefore subject to sampling error; nor can it be related precisely to health Regions, though we have attempted to do so. It also reflects a number of factors which may not be relevant to the NHS, while excluding some which are. In spite of these defects, the Survey suffices to give a broad indication of the orders of magnitude involved. Two main conclusions can be drawn. First, labour costs generally are very substantially higher in the Thames Regions than in the rest of the country. Second, there appear to be some significant differences in labour costs generally between the different provincial Regions. It is also more than likely that variations between different Regions may conceal even wider variations within those Regions – for example, labour costs in inner-city areas are likely to be greater than those in the outlying suburban or rural localities. But the difficulties of measuring these variations reliably from sample data obviously increase when smaller geographical areas are examined.

2.34 The data problems are such that any weighting factor derived from the limited information available could not be recommended with any degree of confidence. The evidence does, however, suggest that cost differentials for and within the Thames Regions are almost certainly significantly greater than those which are attributable to the effect of London Weighting on pay which must in any event be taken into account. **We recommend, as a matter of some urgency, that a detailed study should be undertaken to establish the scale and significance of geographic market cost differences and their effect on the provision of services at Regional and sub-Regional level. In the meantime we also recommend that**

i. London Weighting should continue to be taken into account in determining target allocations and

ii. the probability that the London Weighting adjustment does not fully compensate for market variations should be taken into account subjectively in determining the rate at which actual allocations should be adjusted in relation to target allocations in the Thames RHAs.

PROGRESS TOWARDS REVENUE TARGETS FOR RHAs

Need for Constraints

2.35 A comparison of the revenue target allocations arrived at as described earlier in this chapter with the revenue actually allocated to each RHA in the previous year will reveal how far each RHA is from achieving its target. The histogram in Chapter VI (Figure VI-1) demonstrates the orders of magnitude involved. We consider these large disparities to be indefensible and that they should be removed. But we recognise that this can sensibly only be achieved over a period of time. There are practical limits to the amount of reduction which any RHA could sustain in any one year – particularly in view of the need to remedy the deprivation which exists in some parts of all Regions. Conversely, there are limits beyond which individual RHAs could not, with efficiency and effectiveness, accommodate an unprecedentedly high growth rate. Moreover, it is questionable whether, in a situation in which some RHAs might have little or no growth, a few RHAs should enjoy very high growth.

2.36 In our Interim Report we expressed our support for the phasing out of special protection for the revenue consequences of capital schemes (RCCS), but recommended its continuation for 1976/77 only in a modified form. Ministers subsequently accepted that recommendation whilst at the same time announcing their intention that from 1977/78 onwards RCCS should no longer be protected. RHAs will from now on themselves have to plan their capital investment with regard to the likely availability of revenue. We are fully in sympathy with this decision, which is consistent with the views expressed in our earlier Report, and therefore make no further recommendation on this subject.

Basic Distributional Method

2.37 Under the distributional method adopted for 1976/77 following our Interim Report, those RHAs which were above their revenue targets were held in a standstill position under a 'floor' rule set at zero. The remaining RHAs were brought upwards so far as possible towards parity with each other, subject to a 'ceiling' rule limiting the extent of growth in any one RHA over the previous year to 4% excluding the effects of RCCS. There are disadvantages in continuing this approach. Its application over a period of years would mean progress in some needy RHAs was extremely slow, and in others highly variable, with a large increase in one year followed by much smaller increases subsequently. It is highly sensitive to the level of constraints set to the operation of the formula on the RHAs at the extremes; in some circumstances it can operate in such a way that most RHAs receive the same level of increase, irrespective of variations in their needs; in others, its effect is to permit the very situation deplored in paragraph 2.35, where a few RHAs receive high growth and others, also needy, little or none. Similarly, although the recommendations in our Interim Report relating to floors were not followed in the sense that reductions were not made in allocations to above-target RHAs, the application of a common negative floor to all such RHAs would have taken no account of their relative distances from targets. A continuation of this approach would clearly be inequitable in succeeding years.

2.38   The disadvantages of continuing the 1976/77 method can be avoided by the adoption of a different approach, which is both more sensitive to individual need and more practical in its application. Figure II-5 compares the two approaches. **We recommend that, subject to the constraints outlined in the following paragraphs, changes in the amount of revenue money allocated to RHAs should be in proportion to their distance from target.**

National Growth Rate – 'Floors' and 'Ceilings'
2.39   Target levels are affected by two factors: the extent to which RHAs' relative requirements are already being met according to the criteria applied, and the amount of revenue money available for distribution. The first determines how RHAs stand in relation to each other. The combination with the second determines their distance from target. When there is an increase in revenue nationally, the effect is to raise each RHA's target level. Those who are below target have further to go in order to reach their target; conversely, those who are above target have less far to go. Even if all above-target RHAs were held in a permanent standstill position, with no cuts, the target would eventually catch up with them as national resources increased. If cuts were imposed on the above-target RHAs, the rate at which this happened would be accelerated. Thus change occurs at a rate determined partly by the extent of redistribution it is decided to adopt and partly by the changes in overall resource availability. This interaction must be borne in mind in considering what constraints should be applied to the operation of the revenue distribution system.

2.40   The operation of the proposed distributional method must be constrained in such a way as to secure that, at one extreme, growth or, at the other, cuts do not exceed what is practicable and desirable in the interests of providing an economic and efficient service to patients. In our Interim Report we recommended the application of 'floors' and 'ceilings' to limit the pace of change, and illustrated a range of options showing their operation

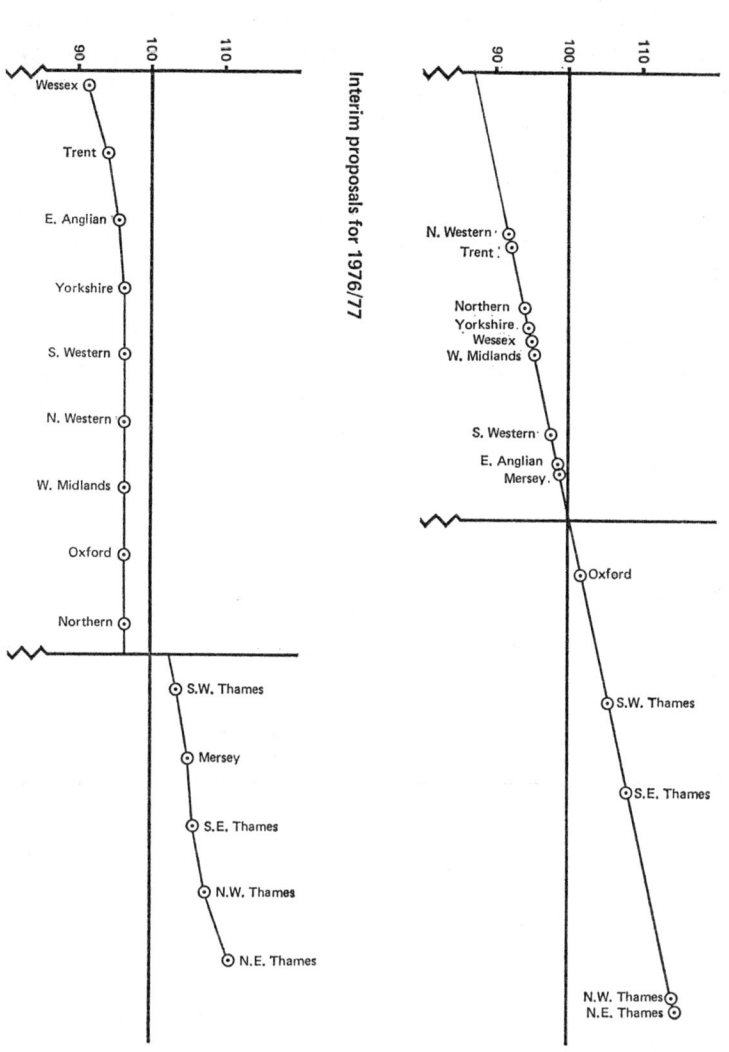

Figure II-5 Charts comparing interim and revised proposals for distributing revenue funds

Revised proposals

Interim proposals for 1976/77

31

at different levels. Since, however, the level at which 'floors' and 'ceilings' should be set depends on the national growth rate, we do not feel able to recommend any single level of 'floor' or 'ceiling' which would be appropriate to all situations which are likely to be encountered in practice. Nevertheless we can suggest certain guiding principles which can be observed in relation to possible variations in national growth rates.

2.41 It is generally accepted that the resources available to the NHS need to grow at a rate of 1% per annum in order to accommodate the increasing cost effects of demographic change, eg the increasing proportion of elderly in the population. Demographic change is of course reflected in the proposed formula (albeit approximately two years in arrear) and in consequence affects both the level at which the target allocation for each RHA is set and its distance from it. Using 1% growth rate as a reference level it is possible to indicate how 'floors' and 'ceilings' might be treated in different national growth rate situations. Four possibilities are considered:

National Growth Rate at
    A. Above 1%
    B. 1%
    C. Zero
    D. Negative.

2.42 The practical options available at each of these four levels of national growth are:

National Growth Rate	Above-Target RHAs	Below-Target RHAs
A—Above 1%	(1) Differential reductions in allocations. (2) Standstill. (3) Differential growth if available resource exceeds that which can be allocated to below-target Regions under the ceiling rule.	Differential growth as recommended in paragraph 2.38.
B—1%	(1) Differential reductions in allocations. (2) Standstill.	Differential growth as recommended in paragraph 2.38.
C—Zero	(1) Differential reductions in allocations. (2) Standstill.	(1) Standstill. (2) Differential growth if allocations to above-target Regions are reduced.
D—Negative	(1) Differential reductions in allocations.	(1) Differential reductions in allocations. (2) Standstill. (3) Limited differential growth.

Setting the Floor

2.43 In situations A and B above, the crucial decision is whether reductions or a standstill should be applied to above-target RHAs. A reduction would cause the RHAs concerned to accommodate the effect of demographic change by redeploying resources *in addition* to the redeployment necessary to assist deprived AHAs within those RHAs. Reduction would probably not be appropriate if, under A, the national growth rate were well in excess of the 1% postulated. Indeed at high growth rates differential growth to even above-target RHAs would not be inappropriate. We take the view, however, that in the event that a decision to reduce allocations to above-target RHAs is taken, the reduction should not exceed 1% in the RHA furthest above its target and should be differentiated proportionately to RHAs at lower levels. **We recommend accordingly.**

2.44 In situation C, whilst it is possible to consider a standstill in all RHAs, it would be contrary to the policy of equalisation and would bear more heavily on the below-target RHAs who would not have the resources available to cope even with the effects of demographic change. Nor would a 'floor' of -1% maximum in the above-target RHAs free sufficient resources to overcome this problem in the others. **In these circumstances, we recommend that consideration should be given to setting the 'floor' at a lower level than -1%.**

2.45 In situation D, similarly, the 'floor' would need to be set at a level lower than -1%, the actual level depending on the reduction in national growth. The aim should, we consider, be to set the 'floor' at the lowest level which could be tolerated at the maximum, probably $-2\frac{1}{2}\%$, in such a way that the RHA furthest below its target might at worst be enabled to stand still at zero growth, differentiated cuts being applied between the two extremes.

2.46 In each case the decision should be influenced by consideration of the possible effect of market cost variations as discussed in paragraphs 2.30 – 2.34.

Setting the Ceiling

2.47 In situations A and B and possibly C above it is necessary to ensure that no RHA receives an increase above that which it could sensibly absorb in a single year. In view of the general considerations of equity outlined above, **we recommend that the operation of the distributional method should be constrained in such a way as to preclude an increase of more**

than 5% over the previous year's allocations in any one RHA. Any revenue in excess of that level should be redistributed to other RHAs in proportion to their distance from target. The level of 5% takes account both of the cessation of RCCS protection and the increased flexibility between capital and revenue, a subject dealt with at greater length elsewhere in this Report.

The Need for Consistency in the Approach

2.48   In framing our recommendations above we have had very much in mind that progress towards target should be a smooth process avoiding harsh accelerations or braking on the way. Radical changes cannot be achieved in a short time; they have to be carefully planned and must be subject to difficult and often protracted local consultations. This is particularly true for the above-target RHAs. If policy decisions are likely to be in the direction of requiring reductions to be made in the allocations to these RHAs, it is in our view far better that this should be established as early as possible and plenty of time allowed for the RHAs to respond. We realise that this may be difficult bearing in mind the uncertainties at present surrounding the future national economic situation. We believe, nonetheless, that an equitable distribution of resources will be easier to achieve if longer range policy objectives on resource allocations can be clearly stated in planning assumptions. This applies to all RHAs and we hope that this point will be kept in mind.

CONCLUSIONS AND SUMMARY OF RECOMMENDATIONS

2.49   In this chapter we have discussed the availability and relevance of indicators of the needs of the population served by a RHA for revenue in the context of particular services. We have recommended which indicators should be used for revenue allocation purposes, and have set out how they can be combined to form a single index of the revenue needs of the population served by each RHA, identified by methods which we have also described. We have drawn attention to the need to take account of cost differences and the means now existing for doing so. Finally, we have set out our views on the need for equity to be achieved as rapidly as possible and the practical constraints on the pace of change, and have established ground rules for progress towards parity. The recommendations contained in this chapter can be summarised as follows:

Assessment of Relative Need for Health Care

2.49.1   **Population** in terms of numbers of people in each Region should be the first criterion of relative need (paragraph 2.2).

34

2.49.2 **The age and sex structure** of each Region's population should be taken into account by means of appropriate national utilisation rates for each of the services specified in this chapter except Ambulances and FPC Administration (paragraphs 2.4, 2.18, 2.20, 2.21, 2.22, 2.23 and 2.27).

2.49.3 **Mortality in the form of SMRs** for each Region should be introduced into the population weightings as a proxy for morbidity on a condition-specific basis for non-psychiatric hospital in-patient services and on an overall basis for non-psychiatric day- and out-patient services, for community health services and for ambulance services (paragraphs 2.15, 2.18, 2.20 and 2.21).

2.49.4 **Fertility rates** for each Region should be introduced into the SMR calculations for the acute general hospital in-patient services in respect of those conditions associated with pregnancy (paragraph 2.15).

2.49.5 **Marital status** should be taken into account in the national utilisation rates applied within each Region to the mental illness in-patient services (paragraph 2.24).

2.49.6 **Patient flows** including where appropriate agency arrangements and extra-territorial management arrangements should be reflected where possible into each weighted population – both numbers and costs – and RHAs should be compensated for the old long-stay patients resident in mental illness or mental handicap hospitals (paragraphs 2.17, 2.18, 2.19, 2.20, 2.26 and 2.27).

2.49.7 **Crude population alone** should be used to determine the relative need for FPC administrative expenditure (paragraph 2.22).

2.49.8 **Caseload** as a separate element in the formula should be abandoned (paragraph 2.28).

2.49.9 **Weighted populations** should be aggregated on the basis of relative expenditure nationally on the services concerned, and the revenue available for services nationally shall be distributed in proportion to each RHA's aggregated weighted population (paragraph 2.29).

2.49.10 **London Weighting** should be taken into account; and pending research on other cost differences between Regions their probable effect should be kept in view in determining the pace of change (paragraph 2.34).

Progress towards RHA Revenue Targets
2.49.11 **Distance from target** should form the basis of the distributional method for revenue (paragraphs 2.37 and 2.38).

2.49.12 **'Ceilings' and 'floors'** should be set to constrain the operation of this distributional method (paragraphs 2.39 – 2.47).

CHAPTER III Distribution of Revenue to Area Health Authorities and Districts

INTRODUCTION

3.1 The criteria for establishing Regional differentiation of need and the methods recommended for resolving the ensuing disparities would have no purpose unless applied to allocations below Regional level. Indeed the only way in which our recommendations can have a real effect is to carry them through to the point where services are actually provided – the Areas and Districts.

3.2 The problems are similar but with significant differences. Few Areas and Districts are entirely self-sufficient. Nearly all provide services of one sort or another to others and many will have to continue to do so for some considerable time. Movements of patients and services across Area and District boundaries occur to a greater extent than across Regional boundaries. Factors which can be largely ignored at Regional level – eg seasonal demands, and the effects of commuter traffic on services – assume far greater significance at sub-Regional level. But the needs of populations served by Areas and Districts remain and are assessable, whatever the variations which occur in delivery of services. And no matter whether these variations are unplanned and unacceptable or planned and acceptable they remain susceptible to treatment in much the same way as their Regional counterparts.

3.3 The same principles recommended for allocations to RHAs can and should therefore in our view be applied to allocations below Regional level. Only the emphasis and the methods need adjusting to suit the sub-Regional context:

3.3.1 As at Regional level, the first step is to establish a revenue target for each locality by methods similar to those applied between RHAs. It is clearly vital that targets should be established on a compatible basis throughout the country. There would be little point in using one basis for remedying disparities between RHAs if RHAs were free to distribute finance to their AHAs (and AHAs to Districts) using different and incompatible criteria. This could actually widen disparities between neighbouring AHAs and Districts in different Regions. Differences will and should of course continue to exist between localities within as well as between RHAs, but these should only be as a result of planning decisions taken within the framework of compatible allocation systems.

3.3.2 Once revenue targets have been set, it has to be decided where each locality stands in relation to its target. This is more difficult within than between RHAs, since expenditure incurred by RHAs and AHAs on behalf of AHAs and Districts has to be taken into account as well as the direct expenditure by the AHAs and Districts.

3.3.3 Finally, it has to be decided how fast each locality can and should move from its starting position as established under 3.3.2 towards its revenue target under 3.3.1. It is not the case that the constraints on progress towards the target can or should be the same in all places. So long as the general trend is in the right direction Authorities should be free to adopt those routes towards the common goal which best suit local circumstances. The pace of movement towards target will depend among other things on the rate at which financial resources can be effectively deployed in real terms or real resources can be redeployed given different local staffing and recruitment situations and different potential for opening, closing or changing the use or condition of local buildings and equipment. Priorities and strategies for service development will also influence choices about where deprivation should be relieved first.

SETTING AHA AND DISTRICT REVENUE TARGETS

Sum to be Distributed

3.4 Revenue targets for RHAs are arrived at in the national formula by distributing the money available *in the allocation year* in accordance with the revenue allocation formula. The counterpart of this approach below Regional level would be to distribute on a formula basis the *actual* Regional allocation for the year. This approach has two main disadvantages:

3.4.1 Since allocations to RHAs are not known until fairly late in the financial year preceding the year of allocation, notional allocations to AHAs and Districts could not be derived until a date too late for them to be fully effective.

3.4.2 Until equality had been achieved between RHAs the use of actual RHA allocations as a basis for sub-Regional targets would lead to the establishment of different targets for AHAs which on national criteria ought to have the same target. One consequence of this would be that some AHAs which should, on national criteria, be shown as being below target could in the Regional context be shown as above target and the converse.

3.5 These difficulties can be overcome by using the *RHA's revenue target* in the current year (ie the year before the allocation year) as the basis of assessing targets for AHAs and Districts. The sum would be known from the outset and would produce revenue targets for AHAs which were equitable in national terms, and the line drawn between AHAs which stood to gain and those which stood to lose would relate to the AHA's position in the national rather than the Regional context. Similarly District targets should be based on AHA revenue targets. **We recommend that AHA target allocations should be calculated from the RHA target allocation and similarly District targets from the AHA target allocations.**

Build-up of Revenue Targets for AHAs
3.6 Since Areas are the sum of their Districts, and there may be wide variations between Districts within Areas, the logical way of formulating AHA targets is, in our view, by an aggregation of District targets. RHAs should therefore begin their assessment of the needs of AHAs by an analysis and then a summation of the needs of the individual Districts within each Area. In this way, AHAs and Districts will have the assurance that particular local problems are not being overlooked. Since the information to be used, and the methods adopted, should be the same whether RHAs are establishing District targets in order to arrive at AHA targets, or whether AHAs are doing so as a starting point in the process of allocation to Districts, the District target should be the same in each case.

3.7 Thus the process of arriving at AHA including District targets must be one in which responsibility is shared by the RHA and AHA. But this co-operative approach in no way alters the quite separate responsibilities of each Authority to decide the actual allocations to an AHA or District as the case may be. A special responsibility rests upon the AHA to ensure that information relevant to the setting of targets is made available to the RHA. Similarly, RHA information should always be at the AHA's disposal. **We recommend that AHA revenue targets should be formulated by aggregation of District revenue targets and that RHAs and AHAs should operate jointly in this process.**

Method of Arriving at Revenue Targets

3.8 Whilst the methods applied nationally in determining RHA revenue targets should in principle be applied to AHA and District targets some modifications need to be made to take account of differences in scale; they fall into two groups:

3.8.1 *Changes necessitated in population weighting by the size of the population involved.* Fewer age/sex bands would have to be used: preliminary study of comparative figures indicates that this would result in insignificant changes. Condition-specific SMRs can be used at Area and District level with some loss of reliability due to the smaller numbers involved. Sensitivity tests indicate, however, that the results will still be closer in most cases to the notionally 'correct' result than would be the case if a cruder measure, such as overall SMRs, were applied. As time goes by and the data base is built up from the $1\frac{3}{4}$ years used initially to the 10 recommended for eventual use, reliability will improve.

3.8.2 *The need for better information.* In national calculations of RHA targets particular aspects of care can safely be assumed to balance out or lack significance in relation to population at Regional level; but this assumption does not necessarily hold good for sub-Regional targets. In particular, attention is drawn to the crucial importance of correct assessment and costing of patient flows between Districts, both for in-patients and for out-patients. Research into the extent of these flows must be carried out at local level, but should proceed from central impetus and guidance. Where out-patients are concerned, the opportunity should be taken to strengthen the information available on use of these services nationally by men and women of different ages. At the same time central information must be produced on specialty costs in suitable groupings. If patient flow adjustments are to give adequate recognition to the burden borne by Districts giving care to people living in other Districts, they must reflect the best possible estimate of the costs nationally of Regional and sub-Regional specialties and not merely of broad categories of care.

We recommend that the revenue targets for sub-Regional levels should be arrived at by applying the same methods as those applied nationally in determining RHA revenue targets subject to the modifications set out above.

Interpretation of Revenue Targets

3.9 It is, however, recognised that targets set by the above method take no account of expenditure incurred by one AHA/District on behalf of others which do not entail patient flows, eg laundry services, nor do they make any allowance for the extra costs of maintaining 'centres of excellence' of one sort or another, including research and development activity, the benefits of which are expected to extend beyond the District in which they are provided. An adjustment for the first category can be made when comparing revenue targets with the starting position. The second category cannot at present be dealt with in this way, and must therefore become a factor to be considered when determining the progress which can and should be made towards target. Authorities will also need to bear in mind the real but unquantifiable impact upon the services they provide of deprivation in its wider social sense. It is conceivable that a particular AHA or District would always be maintained at a level above its indicated target, and that, correspondingly, others would never reach theirs.

3.10 Too rigid an interpretation ought not, in our view, to be placed upon revenue targets assessed on the lines recommended. They nevertheless provide an objective yardstick of relative disparity against which the need for resources, and therefore, the crucial allocation process, can be determined. In the final analysis, judgement must play a considerable part, and it is, therefore, important that there should be open discussion between RHAs, AHAs and DMTs on the way in which targets need to be interpreted in relation to allocations.

COMPARISON OF ACTUAL POSITION WITH TARGETS

3.11 Once revenue targets have been established, the next step is to determine how far each District's resource requirement has already been achieved. This cannot be done simply by comparing the target allocation with that actually received by each District. Since District targets are based on the whole of a RHA's target, the whole of the RHA's actual allocation for services in the current year must be used for comparison, if like is to be compared with like. But the whole RHA allocation is not parcelled out to Districts. Part of it is spent at Regional, and part at Area level. Some of the money spent by RHAs and AHAs goes on specific services to particular Districts. Examples are senior medical staff salaries, CHC expenses and contractual arrangements for hospital services. This expenditure is clearly part of the resources of the Districts concerned, and should be included in an assessment of their actual resources.

3.12 A modest proportion of the RHA allocation is spent at RHA or AHA level in ways which preclude attribution to Districts on a user basis.

Examples are administrative costs. This expenditure should be apportioned to Districts on a notional basis. The Working Party has no strong views on the form this should take. Possible bases are crude or weighted population, or indeed relative spending. What matters is not the method but the fact of apportionment, which should be accompanied by a clear statement from the RHA (or AHA) on the basis of their figuring. AHAs would then have a solid foundation for discussing with RHAs and DMTs with AHAs not only the reasons for any disparities between their revenue targets and the money and services actually received, but the merits of the current balance between money and services and the policy to be adopted in future.

3.13 A further factor to be taken into account is, as mentioned above, the provision made in certain Districts for services to other Districts which do not entail patient flows, such as centralised laundry services or pathology services provided at a supra-District level. Where these services are dealt with on a cross-accounting basis, the costs and benefits to the Districts involved will be available. In any case, the net cost to each District from such services should be included in the assessment of actual resources to ensure that comparisons are made on a realistic basis.

3.14 **Thus we recommend that the assessment of the actual resources of each District for comparison with target should comprise four elements:**
   i. **the final allocation in the District in the current year, less any money allocated to the District from the RHA's Service Increment For Teaching (since money for the SIFT is excluded from the target calculation),**
   ii. **expenditure by the RHA or AHA on specific services to the District, apportioned on a user basis,**
   iii. **a notional share of any remaining expenditure by the RHA and AHA,**
   iv. **the net cost arising from supra-District provision of services not entailing patient flows.**

3.15 Comparison between the actual resources so assessed and the target will give some indication of the direction and degree of change to be aimed at. Figure III.1 illustrates the process.

PROGRESS TOWARDS REVENUE TARGETS FOR AHAs AND DISTRICTS

3.16 This then is the starting point for action when the revenue allocations are known for the following year. If the total RHA allocation reveals that funds are available for development, it may be possible to have some growth

42

Figure III-1

Comparison of Revenue Shares and Targets

District notional revenue requirements based on apportionment of total RHA revenue target (less SIFT)

Current District revenue share based on apportionment of total RHA revenue allocation

District A revenue target based on modified national method allowing for costed patient flows.

Notional RHA apportionment
Specific RHA services
Notional AHA apportionment
Specific AHA services
Final allocation for District A including the costs of services provided by other Districts for District A *less* (i) any SIFT and (ii) costs of providing services for other Districts.

District B revenue target based on modified national method allowing for costed patient flows. (District B is a single-District Area.)

Notional RHA apportionment
Specific RHA services
Final allocation for District B including the costs of services provided by other Districts for District B *less* (i) any SIFT and (ii) costs of providing services for other Districts. (This includes AHA services as District B is a single-District Area.)

in all AHAs/Districts. Nevertheless a major proportion of these funds will no doubt be allocated to the more deprived AHAs/Districts to enable the services to be built up, having regard to the distance from target of each AHA or District revealed by the comparison described above but bearing in mind that total self-sufficiency in every AHA and District is not an immediate or necessarily even a longer-term aim. If a cut-back in total terms is required in the following year these cuts will no doubt fall more heavily upon the near or above-target AHAs/Districts. 'Floors' and 'ceilings' on the national pattern are not applicable below Regional level, where very much wider variation may be possible due to closure or opening of major facilities. The planning of developments and cuts is for discussion at Regional, Area and District level, with regard to the impact of local considerations on the pace of change. **We so recommend.** Points which should be borne in mind in this discussion include:

3.16.1 Special local factors, such as the extent to which alternative facilities relieve or add to pressure on the NHS.

3.16.2 Abnormal workloads, which are not fully reflected in the estimates.

3.16.3 The revenue consequences of capital developments coming on stream.

3.16.4 Capacity to absorb revenue change in terms of capital stock and manpower. This may pose particular problems in RHAs where the need for change is concentrated in one or two AHAs.

3.16.5 Planning considerations – need to develop priority services, planned closures or changes of use, policy decisions whether or not to alter present patterns for delivery of care and the consequential patient flows, policy decisions on the extent to which it may be desirable to create or maintain 'centres of excellence'.

3.16.6 The need to hold reserves – though these should be kept to a minimum in order to secure the most equitable distribution possible and should be concentrated wherever possible at the AHA or District.

3.17 The proposals outlined in this chapter should enable Health Authorities to determine allocations in accordance with common criteria and a common methodology while allowing necessary flexibility to meet local variation. *It is stressed that this approach can work only if the criteria and methods of allocation are made aboslutely clear to those receiving the allocations at all levels in the NHS, and that there should be continuing discussion between all concerned as part of an ongoing process of clarification and improvement.*

CONCLUSIONS AND SUMMARY OF RECOMMENDATIONS

3.18 In this chapter we have drawn attention to the crucial importance of carrying the principles of revenue allocation used nationally through to the allocation of revenue to AHAs and Districts. We have set out the points at which the methods and criteria adopted can be the same or similar at the different levels, and the points at which they must diverge. We have stated our belief that it is possible to establish a common methodology across the country for achieving equality and have described the steps enabling targets to be produced and compared with the current position. Local factors of a practical nature must be taken into account in the interpretation of progress towards targets, and we have suggested mechanisms enabling this to occur. The recommendations in this chapter can be summarised as follows:

3.18.1 **The whole of each RHA's revenue target** should form the basis of the notional distribution to determine District allocations (paragraph 3.5).

3.18.2 **AHA revenue targets** should be determined by aggregating the District targets (paragraph 3.7).

3.18.3 **District targets** should be formulated by co-operation between AHAs and RHAs (paragraph 3.7).

3.18.4 **National methods** for arriving at RHA targets should be applied as nearly as possible in the sub-Regional context (paragraph 3.8).

3.18.5 **Actual resources** should be adjusted in certain ways in order to allow a valid comparison to be made with the targets (paragraphs 3.11 – 3.15).

3.18.6 **Pace of change** in the sub-Regional context must take account of local considerations (paragraph 3.16).

CHAPTER IV   Additional NHS Service
Costs Arising from the
Clinical Teaching of
Medical and Dental
Students

DEFINITIONS AND DISTINCTIONS

4.1 The NHS has a statutory responsibility to make available to the Medical Schools of the Universities clinical facilities for the teaching of medical and dental students. The University Grants Committee is responsible for providing the direct costs of their education. These clinical facilities are mainly provided in designated 'teaching hospitals' but for allocation purposes account needs to be taken of all premises providing such facilities whether designated or not. The term 'teaching hospital' is used in this wider context in this Report.

4.2 Teaching hospitals are on average more costly to run than hospitals in which no teaching takes place. But, as we pointed out in Chapter I, the incidence of these higher costs bears no relationship either to the size or needs of the populations served by these hospitals. Thus means must be found of identifying the additional costs *necessarily incurred* as a direct result of the NHS's commitment to provide clinical facilities, protecting the finance involved from the effect of allocation processes based upon population and service need criteria, as recommended in Chapters II and III, and arranging for its allocation on an equitable and proportionate basis to the institutions discharging the commitment.

4.3 The higher cost of teaching hospitals is not wholly and directly attributable to the teaching function and the presence of students. Factors also contributing to higher cost levels include:

4.3.1 Regional specialties tend to be located in teaching hospitals.

4.3.2 Research work tends also to be similarly concentrated.

4.3.3 Over the years teaching hospitals in various degrees have developed as 'centres of excellence'.

4.4 In our Interim Report and as an interim measure for 1976/77 only, we recommended a 'Teaching and Research Allowance'. The use of this title led to some misunderstanding and questions were raised as to the degree of protection it afforded to the factors mentioned above. We must make it clear at the outset that *the sole purpose of the 'allowance' which we later propose is to cover the additional service costs incurred by the NHS in providing facilities for the clinical teaching of medical and dental students.* Its purpose is to provide an increment to service costs. We believe this will be better understood if it were referred to as a 'Service Increment for Teaching – SIFT' and we have adopted this terminology in this Report.

4.5 The question has been posed how are the additional costs of teaching hospitals referred to in 4.3 above to be financed if not through SIFT? Clearly these factors have strong associations with the teaching function but by no means exclusively. Many Regional specialties and much research work are to be found in non-teaching hospitals, many of which have developed as 'centres of excellence' in their own right. Whilst it may be found convenient and, in many cases, highly beneficial to regard teaching hospitals as natural centres in which to conduct research and provide higher standards of care, this ought in our view to continue to be a question of choice to be exercised by Health Authorities in consultation with the other interests concerned.

4.6 It has to be recognised too that, since the resources available to the NHS are finite, a balance has to be struck between the desirability and need to pursue excellence on the one hand and the need to provide generally better standards of provision and care. There is no escaping the fact that one centre's 'excellence' may be bought at the price of another's 'deprivation'. We stress that this is not an argument against excellence, which we support, but for a conscious balance to be struck in the way limited resources are deployed. It is our view that such deployment should be judged in relation to the needs of the populations served and therefore that the factors to which we have referred fall to be considered and dealt with within the main service allocation to RHAs, AHAs and Districts.

4.7 The interaction of these factors (paragraph 4.3 above) on the higher costs of teaching hospitals is, we have found, difficult to interpret and quantify from data currently available. It is also possible that part of the disparities between RHAs is explicable in these terms. Research into the interrelationship between 'centres of excellence', centres for clinical teaching and centres where other educational and research facilities are concentrated to establish their effect upon the level of service provision and their impact upon costs should, in our view, be undertaken. **We recommend accordingly.**

IDENTIFYING THE SERVICE INCREMENT
FOR TEACHING (SIFT)

4.8   In our Interim Report, we used the known historic 'excess' costs of the teaching hospitals formerly administered by Boards of Governors as a basis for calculating the recommended teaching and research allowance to be protected in the 1976/77 allocations. London and provincial teaching hospitals were treated separately and this gave rise to two levels of allowance. The differential treatment accorded attracted widespread criticism. We accept the force of this criticism. Since all medical schools and their associated teaching hospitals produce graduates acceptable to the examining bodies, there are, prima facie, no grounds justifying a wide differential in cost. We have therefore sought a method which would provide a common basis for determining and distributing an allowance for SIFT as from 1977/78.

The Basic Calculation

4.9   The starting point is to establish the extent to which the costs of teaching hospitals are known to exceed those of non-teaching hospitals and relate them to the numbers of students undergoing clinical teaching. For this purpose we have used the latest costing data available, namely those relating to 1973/74, and have revalued them to a March 1975 price base. This is convenient for comparison with our interim proposals for 1976/77. We have also included the costs of the teaching hospitals administered by the former Newcastle Board of Governors. The observable excess costs of these teaching hospitals are shown in Table IV-1.

4.10   As a baseline for determining the 'excess cost' we have used the '45 Sample Hospital Formula' devised by the Department for assessing the revenue costs of new hospitals. It is important to remember that this formula produces a level of cost higher than the average costs of all non-teaching hospitals. It is, therefore, an objective not an attained level of funding. Its use for the purpose of determining 'excess' costs of teaching hospitals assumes that the service costs of these hospitals are at the objective level. This is important in interpreting the results shown in Table IV-1.

4.11   The median 'excess cost per student' is seen to lie between two London teaching hospitals – the London Hospital and University College Hospital. The wide discrepancies to be found below the median are, we consider, not attributable to differences in the *additional* costs of providing clinical facilities. They are much more likely to be explained by the fact that average service

Table IV-1   **Summary of Calculations to Derive 1973/74 Excess Costs per Student in Former Teaching Hospital Groups**

£000s at March 1975 Prices

Former Teaching Hospital Groups	Estimated Relevant Costs 1973/74	Baseline Service Costs	Excess Costs 1 – 2	Number of Students 1975/76	Excess Cost per Student
	1	2	3	4	5
Westminster	13,310	9,300	4,010	210	19.1
Charing Cross	10,790	7,190	3,600	200	18.0
Oxford	13,290	10,820	2,470	140	17.6
St. Thomas'	13,870	9,130	4,740	280	16.9
Royal Free	10,170	6,250	3,920	250	15.7
St. George's	10,270	7,550	2,720	200	13.6
St. Mary's	12,170	8,920	3,250	300	10.8
St. Bart's	9,600	6,550	3,050	290	10.5
Kings College	14,520	11,370	3,150	310	10.2
London	12,870	9,670	3,200	330	9.7
Median					9.5
University College	10,930	8,240	2,690	290	9.3
Middlesex	9,830	7,210	2,620	300	8.7
Guy's	12,950	9,770	3,180	390	8.2
Liverpool	12,400	10,330	2,070	260	8.0
Bristol	11,800	9,340	2,460	320	7.7
Birmingham	15,110	12,580	2,530	420	6.0
Manchester	11,910	10,140	1,770	340	5.2
Sheffield	13,300	11,840	1,460	290	5.0
Leeds	9,840	8,910	930	240	3.9
Newcastle	8,480	7,550	930	280	3.3
Totals/Average	237,410	182,660	54,750	5,640	9.7

NOTES:

Col 1. Excluding London Weighting and adjusted for UGC funding (paragraphs 4.16 – 4.18).

Col 2. Based on '45 Sample Hospital Formula' data (paragraph 4.10) applied to the workload and specialty mix of the teaching hospital groups.

Col 3. Notional numbers of students (based on UGC forecasts for two years ahead of 1973/74) undergoing clinical teaching in hospital groups, dental students being counted at ¼ (paragraphs 4.23 – 4.27 and 4.29).

costs in these hospitals fall below the level indicated by the '45 Sample Hospital Formula'. The Department's experience in comparing the formula calculation of the revenue consequences of capital development at many of these hospitals with their existing revenue costs confirms this view. Thus if it were possible to correct for the lower level of service provision, the notional 'excess costs' of these hospitals would be likely to approach the median.

4.12 At the other end of the scale, the much higher excess cost per student in some of the London hospitals may well be explicable in terms of the extent to which these hospitals have developed as 'centres of excellence' rather than that the additional service costs of teaching are necessarily that much higher.

4.13 We have concluded that the median excess cost per student can justifiably be taken as the starting point for calculating the sum to be protected as a SIFT. The median could either be the median hospital or the median student. We have taken the former; erring if at all therefore on the generous side.

4.14 It has to be borne in mind, however, that the median cannot be said to be a precise measure of the justifiable excess cost for the purposes of SIFT. Hospitals lying close to the median are clearly recognised as 'centres of excellence' (as indeed are others well below the median). The median therefore includes an element of excellence over and above that implicit in the baseline cost. There are, however, no data available which can be used to identify reliably the 'excellence' element. Indeed comparative unit cost data suggest that much of this element may in fact be traceable to very high unit costs in support rather than clinical services, eg catering, laundry, cleaning, porterage and other ancillary services. We are therefore forced to rely upon the evidence of the York Study which we used in our Interim Report; namely that nationally 75% of the observable additional costs in teaching hospitals may be attributable to the teaching commitment. We take the view that this proportion is likely to be valid at the median even though it would clearly be erroneous at the extremes. We believe, again, that its application would err on the side of generosity.

4.15 **We therefore recommend that 75% of the median excess cost per student calculated as above should be used as the basis for determining the protection within allocations to be afforded through the SIFT.**

Special Factors

4.16 We have examined the costs of London and provincial teaching hospitals in an attempt to identify factors which might explain the wide differences in excess costs and which ought to be taken into account in determining the level of SIFT. Two such factors have emerged:

4.16.1 The lower level of UGC funding of the London medical schools compared with the provincial schools.

4.16.2 Higher unit costs incurred in London, exemplified by London Weighting, but also applicable to other expenditure.

4.17 UGC financial provision for the London medical schools is at a relatively lower level per clinical medical student than in the provinces. The unit cost in 1973/74 (updated to March 1975 price levels) was £2,684 in the provinces and £1,888 in London. The difference of about £800 per student will, we consider, account in part for the relatively lower 'excess' costs in the provinces. The unit costs of the UGC are concerned directly with the costs of academic salaries and with the maintenance of University departments. Even so the difference is, we consider, bound to affect the costs of providing clinical facilities. **We recommend that the Department and the UGC should examine the position. Meanwhile we also recommend that the difference should be taken into account by augmenting the SIFT for the Thames RHAs by an amount of £800 per clinical student.** The figures in Tables IV–1 and IV–2 have been adjusted in this way.

4.18 Examination of the unit and departmental costs of the London teaching hospitals reveals them to be higher than the national average. Clearly one factor at play here is the effect of London Weighting on staff salaries. Adjustments for this still leave large and unexplained differences. We have referred in previous chapters to the probability that economic factors may cause geographical variations in the cost of providing the same level of service, and have recommended further research into this problem. Meanwhile **we recommend that an appropriate allowance for the effect of London Weighting should be added to the SIFT for the Thames RHAs.** The figures in Tables IV–1 and IV–2 have been adjusted in this way.

4.19 For illustrative purposes only, the effect of our recommendations on the costs of the hospital groups used to arrive at a median excess cost per student is shown in Table IV–2.

Table IV-2   **Illustrative Cost Comparison to show Residual Costs not covered by SIFT**

£000s at March 1975 Prices

Former Teaching Hospital Groups	Estimated Relevant Costs 1973/74	Recommended Basis (1975/76)			Residual Excess Costs 1 − 4
		Baseline Service Costs	SIFT based on 1975/76 Students	Total 2+3	
	1	2	3	4	5
Westminster	14,220	10,090	1,790	11,880	+2,340
Charing Cross	11,690	7,800	1,710	9,510	+2,180
Oxford	13,290	10,820	1,000	11,820	+1,470
St Thomas'	14,860	9,910	2,390	12,300	+2,560
Royal Free	10,950	6,780	2,130	8,910	+2,040
St George's	11,000	8,190	1,710	9,900	+1,100
St Mary's	13,100	9,680	2,560	12,240	+ 860
St Bart's	10,370	7,110	2,470	9,580	+ 790
Kings College	15,580	12,340	2,650	14,990	+ 590
London	13,850	10,490	2,820	13,310	+ 540
University College	11,760	8,940	2,470	11,410	+ 350
Middlesex	10,630	7,830	2,560	10,390	+ 240
Guy's	13,980	10,600	3,330	13,930	+ 50
Liverpool	12,400	10,330	1,850	12,180	+ 220
Bristol	11,800	9,340	2,280	11,620	+ 180
Birmingham	15,110	12,580	2,990	15,570	− 460
Manchester	11,910	10,140	2,420	12,560	− 650
Sheffield	13,300	11,840	2,070	13,910	− 610
Leeds	9,840	8,910	1,710	10,620	− 780
Newcastle	8,480	7,550	2,000	9,550	−1,070
Totals	248,120	191,270	44,910	236,180	+11,940

NOTES:

Col 1. Including London Weighting and unadjusted for UGC funding (paragraphs 4.16 – 4.18).

Col 2. Based on '45 Sample Hospital Formula' data (paragraph 4.10) applied to the work-load and specialty mix of the teaching hospital groups, including London Weighting.

Col 3. Based on notional numbers of students including dental at $\frac{1}{4}$ (paragraphs 4.23 – 4.27 and 4.29) plus UGC funding and element of London Weighting appropriate to SIFT.

Col 5. Including an element for London Weighting.

4.20   The spread of residual excess costs shown in the table illustrates the points we have made in paragraphs 4.11 and 4.12 above. It also demonstrates the care which will need to be exercised by Health Authorities in adjusting allocations to the Districts in which teaching hospitals are situated. High standards of care have been carefully built up over many years and are not lightly to be put at risk. Similarly the raising of lower-cost levels of service provision needs careful consideration in relation to other priorities. We return to this subject later.

DETERMINING THE SUMS TO BE PROTECTED THROUGH SIFT AND THE BASIS FOR THEIR DISTRIBUTION

4.21   It is implicit in our approach that the purposes which SIFT is designed to serve are related directly to the numbers of students undergoing clinical teaching. We have had to consider which students should be covered by the protection afforded, what numbers of students should be used for distribution purposes, and how distribution should be handled at each level of allocation.

4.22   Among the observations submitted on our Interim Report was the suggestion that number and grades of staff and the range or number of academic departments may have a greater effect on service costs than student numbers alone. This may be so – and we have considered the point carefully – but we have come to the conclusion that where the cost effect of such factors does not also reflect actual student numbers, it is an effect which SIFT is not designed to cover. Student numbers remain in our view the most satisfactory and equitable basis for assessing and distributing the SIFT.

STUDENTS TO BE INCLUDED

Research Students
4.23   There was no substantial criticism of the approach taken in our Interim Report that research students should be excluded on the grounds that NHS expenditure is not significantly affected by them and their numbers are fairly evenly distributed between Regions. There are considerable practical difficulties in the way of defining 'research students' who are far from being a homogeneous group. The only available figures are of postgraduate students registered for higher degrees and these are expressed as 'whole-time equivalents' since they include many part-time students. Policy varies between departments on whether students register for a higher degree or enter for a Royal College qualification or neither. Whilst we recognise

that the work of some students might have a considerable effect on service costs, most of them have a negligible effect and it can be argued that the contributions which they make to service functions represent a net gain to the NHS. The numbers involved are comparatively small and **we recommend that they should continue to be disregarded for the purposes of SIFT.**

Dental Students

4.24 In our Interim Report we concluded that one-quarter of dental students in clinical training should be added to the medical students for the purpose of calculating and distributing an allowance. This was based upon the fact that dental students receive most of their clinical training in out-patient departments and that expenditure in these departments accounts for one-quarter of teaching hospital expenditure. The method was admittedly crude and has been criticised on the grounds that dental clinical training is mostly in out-patient departments specially equipped and staffed for the purpose and that dental students also receive clinical training in general medicine and surgery.

4.25 It has also been suggested that the services in dental schools are provided solely for the purposes of teaching and incur costs which would otherwise fall to be met by the general dental practitioner services. It is also the case that not all medical schools have associated dental schools and dental hospitals and any error in the adjustment made for dental students could bear more heavily on those which do. We recognise the force of these arguments but we do not feel able to accept, as claimed by some, that the total costs of the clinical departments of dental schools should be directly attributed to the teaching function. To the extent that they discharge a significant service function in cost terms, those costs should be met from the service allocations.

4.26 Those who had reservations about the weighting and others whom we have consulted have been unable to identify or suggest a method of taking dental students into account in which greater confidence could be reposed. Furthermore the median cost per student, recommended as the baseline, includes the costs of dental departments and a change in the weighting for such students would not increase the level of protection afforded nationally through SIFT.

4.27 We have concluded therefore that **we should continue to recommend the weighting of one-quarter for dental students until such time as further study, which we also recommend, can suggest a better basis.**

Determining a National Sum for SIFT

4.28   The method described in the preceding paragraphs is intended only as a basis for determining how much of the total revenue available for distribution to Health Authorities should be protected from the effects of the revenue allocation formula and so provide independently a service increment for teaching. It is not a method which can be used annually because it is based upon the historic costs of selected hospitals and takes no account of the expansion which has already taken place in the numbers of medical students, many of whom receive much of their clinical training in hospitals other than designated teaching hospitals. We understand that this practice is likely to grow. There would in any event be considerable technical difficulties in using the method to recalculate SIFT annually. Fluctuations in student numbers and cost levels would disrupt the pattern of allocations and sensible forward planning. We therefore consider it important that the method should be used only as a basis for arriving at the total sum to be protected and further that this sum should be held constant for the three years 1977/78 to 1979/80, adjusted only for price changes. It should then be reviewed in the light of later cost information and the results of the research which we have elsewhere suggested.

4.29   We have considered whether during the three-year period the national sum should be scaled to take account in each year of the expected annual growth in student numbers. There is, in any event, a need to prepare in advance for major growth; a need which we recognised in our Interim Report by using forecasts of student numbers two years ahead. We have come to the conclusion that the best course would be to fix the national sum for the next three years on the basis of the projected student numbers for 1980/81. **We therefore recommend that nationally the sum to be protected in allocations should be determined by multiplying 75% of the median excess cost per student by the projected number of students for 1980/81 (dental students ranking at one-quarter), to which should be added, in respect of the Thames RHAs, an adjustment for London Weighting and for UGC funding.**

4.30   Application of the above recommendation produces a national SIFT of £72.38 millions (approximate figure at March 1975 prices) calculated as follows:

9,340 students × £7,125 (75% median excess cost per student)
$$= £66.55 \text{ million}$$

plus   £2.52 million London Weighting

plus   £3.31 million UGC funding adjustment

Total national SIFT   £72.38 million

Distributing the National SIFT to RHAs

4.31 The incidence of the additional service costs which SIFT is designed to protect should in equity be directly proportionate to the scale of the teaching activity undertaken. We consider student numbers to be the best indication of this activity and **accordingly recommend that expected student numbers in 1980/81 should be used to distribute SIFT proportionately to RHAs.**

4.32 To avoid marginal fluctuations **we also recommend that the student numbers so used should be rounded up or down to the nearest multiple of five.**

Comparison between Interim (T and R) and Final (SIFT) Proposals

4.33 Table IV–3 applies the recommendations in the foregoing paragraphs to 1977/78 and compares them with the actual teaching and research allowances funded in 1976/77. Although the national sum for SIFT is increased

Table IV–3   **Comparison between T & R Allowance 1976/77 and Proposed SIFT 1977/78**

£000s at March 1975 Prices

Regional Health Authority	1976/77 T & R	1977/78 Proposed SIFT				Differences in Sums Protected
		Basic	London Weighting	UGC Adjustment	Total	
Northern	2,354	3,278			3,278	924
Yorkshire	2,365	3,563			3,563	1,198
Trent	4,664	7,446			7,446	2,782
East Anglian	715	1,283			1,283	568
NW Thames	13,284	8,942	760	999	10,701	−2,583
NE Thames	15,379	10,474	890	1,170	12,534	−2,845
SE Thames	10,411	7,802	663	872	9,337	−1,074
SW Thames	2,808	2,423	206	271	2,900	92
Wessex	1,925	2,779			2,779	854
Oxford	1,320	1,924			1,924	604
S Western	2,211	2,850			2,850	639
W Midlands	3,009	3,883			3,883	874
Mersey	2,750	3,563			3,563	813
N Western	4,868	6,341			6,341	1,473
Totals	68,063	66,551	2,519	3,312	72,382	4,319

(largely as a result of using 1980/81 student numbers), the distribution between RHAs is significantly different. This is to be expected since a common basis has been used to determine the national sum for distribution. The effect of this change has important implications for teaching hospitals, particularly in the Thames RHAs, and particularly in determining allocations to AHAs and Districts. We deal with this point later.

Incorporating SIFT in the Revenue Allocation Formula

4.34   To ensure that the SIFT to RHAs is protected from the redistributional effects of the allocation formula, three steps are necessary:

4.34.1   In determining the target allocation for each RHA, the national SIFT sum must first be deducted from the total revenue available for distribution. The formula then calculates the target service allocation on the remainder.

4.34.2   Similarly the SIFT apportionment to each RHA needs to be deducted from the RHA's starting allocation (ie the previous year's total allocation including T and R for 1976/77) before calculating the differential growth rate to be applied proportionate to each RHA's distance from its target (Chapter II paragraph 2.38).

4.34.3   Finally, the SIFT deducted in 4.34.2 is added back to each RHA's allocation to provide the total (service + SIFT) allocation for the year.

We recommend that this procedure is followed.

4.35   The general effect of the changes proposed for 1977/78 will be twofold. Above-target RHAs receiving less by way of SIFT than they did through T and R allowance in 1976/77 will appear to be further above their service revenue targets. This is because the arrangement proposed above does not directly allow changes in the level of SIFT to reduce the RHA's allocation as a whole. Only if it were decided, for other reasons, actually to reduce the allocation to such RHAs would there be a marginal change. For example, if the service allocation were to be cut by 1%, the effect would be to reduce in addition the difference between the former T and R allowance and the new SIFT by 1%. The effect is negligible therefore and no special arrangement is thought necessary. Below-target RHAs whose SIFT apportionment is higher than the former T and R will also appear to be further below their targets. But from this position they will also attract a higher rate of growth.

4.36   Distribution of SIFT to AHAs and Districts should, in our view, be subject to certain principles and guidelines, viz:

4.36.1   The whole of the SIFT received by RHAs should be distributed to AHAs.

4.36.2   All AHAs and Districts that contribute to undergraduate teaching, whether or not so designated, should receive an appropriate part of the SIFT.

4.36.3   The starting point for distribution to AHAs should be the incidence of the teaching function as measured by the proportionate student load (in whole-time equivalent).

4.36.4   The distribution of the protected sum should be kept in view when determining the total revenue allocation for services which itself needs to make provision for Regional specialties and 'centres of excellence' whether sited in teaching hospitals or elsewhere.

4.36.5   Similar principles should be followed by AHAs in making allocations to Districts, but the need for adjustment will certainly be greater.

4.36.6   Authorities should consult University Liaison Committees before finally determining allocations.

We so recommend.

4.37   In interpreting 4.36.3 above, it would be quite wrong to adhere rigidly to student numbers alone as a basis for distributing the protected sum. Local circumstances may require a more flexible approach, particularly in the case of dental students, and this can only be decided following consultations with local interests concerned. It is true, of course, that if some AHAs or Districts receive a greater proportion of the protected sum than an allocation based solely on student numbers would appear to justify, then other Districts or AHAs will receive a smaller proportion than would seem justified on this basis. The aim should be that the money should be distributed between AHAs, and between Districts, on an equitable basis having regard to all relevant factors. Of these, student numbers will no doubt generally be the most important single factor, but by no means the only one.

4.38   In general, minor changes in expected student numbers should not be used automatically to claim or justify an increase or reduction in the protected sum. In each individual case the question should be asked whether there has been a contraction or expansion in clinical teaching activity affecting NHS costs such as would justify a change in the allocation; and if so, how the change should be reflected.

4.39 In allocations to AHAs and Districts, particular account needs to be taken of the redistributional effect of the changes now recommended. At this level the differences between the former T and R allowance and the new SIFT are very significant. We have deliberately proposed (paragraphs 4.34 and 4.35) that these changes should not directly affect allocations to RHAs in the short term at least. Neither, in our view, should AHA and District allocations be adjusted pro rata and immediately in accordance with the change. The implication of our recommendations in London is that sums which were protected in 1976/77 as directly attributable to teaching are no longer so protected and susceptible therefore to the operation of the revenue formula. In effect they have been transferred to the service allocation. But it has to be recognised that these sums are at present committed to the provision of a certain level of service or indeed a level of excellence and their precipitate withdrawal by RHAs or AHAs would clearly put those services at considerable risk, with consequences that would not, in our view, be in the best interests of the NHS as a whole. We are not saying that current AHA and District allocations should remain inviolate—this would be contrary to the fundamental principle underlying all our recommendations. There is clearly, however, need for considered judgement to be exercised in the pace at which change can be brought about. For this reason **we recommend that AHA and District allocations should not be adjusted solely, proportionately and directly as a consequence of a change in the level of SIFT.** Such adjustments as need to be made in the service allocation for other reasons should be carefully phased to avoid putting important services at risk. We are convinced that this can be done and that the Authorities concerned have evidence available which will assist in determining an appropriate pace of change.

Special Cases

4.40 In our Interim Report we recommended that special protection should be given to two hospitals, Northwick Park and Hammersmith, because of the additional costs they incur arising from their role as national research centres. We do not consider that it would be appropriate for the recommendations we put forward in this chapter to be applied to the special position of these hospitals. The postgraduate hospitals in London, presently administered by preserved Boards of Governors, are in a similar situation.

We recommend that the Department should consider the position of these hospitals separately with the Authorities concerned; as a guideline we would further recommend that, as an interim measure, any special protection provided should not exceed 75% of the excess costs of Northwick Park and Hammersmith Hospitals as compared to the costs of a sample of hospitals of similar size and type. Such an arrangement would be outside the scope of the SIFT proposed in this chapter.

CONCLUSIONS AND SUMMARY OF RECOMMENDATIONS

4.41 In this chapter we have sought to explain why additional service costs necessarily incurred as a result of the presence of medical students need to be the subject of special protection within revenue allocations. We have set out methods of identifying the sum of money involved, and of ensuring that it is taken into account in the revenue distribution process to RHAs, AHAs and Districts. In recommending changes, we have also expounded the mechanism necessary to ensure a smooth transition from old to new. Throughout, we have drawn attention to needs for further research where they exist. Our recommendations can be summarised as follows:

4.41.1 **'Service Increment For Teaching – SIFT'** should be the term used to describe the element within revenue allocations to cover the additional service costs incurred by the NHS in providing facilities for the clinical teaching of medical and dental students (paragraph 4.4).

4.41.2 **Research should be set in hand** on
a. the effects on levels of service provision and costs of (i) 'centres of excellence', (ii) centres for clinical teaching, and (iii) centres where other educational and research facilities are concentrated (paragraph 4.7), and on

b. the basis for taking account of dental students for SIFT purposes (paragraph 4.27).

4.41.3 **75% of the median excess cost per student** of teaching hospitals set against comparable non-teaching hospitals should be the starting point for calculating the sum to be protected as a SIFT (paragraph 4.15).

4.41.4 **Allowance should be made in the SIFT for the Thames RHAs for two special factors:** the lower level of UGC funding of the London medical schools (which should also be examined by the DHSS and the UGC), and the effect of London Weighting (paragraphs 4.17 and 4.18).

4.41.5 **The basis for assessing and distributing the SIFT should remain student numbers** (paragraph 4.22), disregarding research students (paragraph 4.23) and weighting dental students at ¼ (paragraph 4.27).

4.41.6 **Projected student numbers for 1980/81** (paragraph 4.29) should be the basis for fixing the amount of SIFT nationally for the next three years, subject to adjustment for price changes during that period and to review thereafter (paragraph 4.28), and SIFT should be distributed proportionately to RHAs on that basis (paragraph 4.31). The student numbers used for the latter purpose should be rounded up or down to the nearest multiple of five (paragraph 4.32).

4.41.7 **In incorporating SIFT in allocations** it should be deducted from starting allocations and from total revenue in calculating RHAs' service target allocations and differential growth proportionate to distance from target. SIFT should then be added back to each RHA's allocation to provide the total revenue allocation for the year (paragraph 4.34).

4.41.8 **Sub-regionally,** after consultation with University Liaison Committees, all AHAs and Districts that contribute to teaching should receive an appropriate part of the SIFT based on the incidence of the teaching function. Student numbers should be the chief but not the sole criterion (paragraphs 4.36 – 4.38). AHA and District allocations should not be adjusted solely, proportionately and directly as a consequence of a change in the level of SIFT (paragraph 4.39).

4.41.9 **The special position of Northwick Park and Hammersmith Hospitals,** and of the postgraduate hospitals in London, should be considered by the DHSS and the Authorities concerned. As an interim measure any continued special protection for the former two hospitals should not exceed 75% of their excess costs compared with those of a sample of similar hospitals (paragraph 4.40).

CHAPTER V   Capital

BACKGROUND

5.1 The amount, age and quality of the capital stock of the NHS varies both between and within Regions and this variation does not accord with differences in relative need. It has also to be recognised that the NHS is unlikely in the short term to be able to raise its capital investment to the level necessary to meet all possible requirements – to rebuild all old hospitals, to fill all absolute gaps in the services and to correct all imbalances caused by mislocation of capital stock. The resources required to do all these things would be greater by many times than even the peak expenditure on capital in recent years. The task of improving capital stock and achieving a sensible distribution is essentially long-term. The annual capital programme therefore has to be viewed not in the light of what is required in absolute terms, but in the light of what can be afforded. Its distribution must consequently be considered as a means of sharing limited resources on a basis of relative need. But there is no reason why the distributional system should not follow the same logical steps as have already been discussed in relation to revenue – setting capital targets, comparing them with existing facilities and determining the pace at which progress can be made towards the target. The following sections of this chapter discuss these processes: first in relation to allocations to RHAs and then in terms of applying similar principles in the sub-Regional context.

SETTING RHA CAPITAL TARGETS

5.2 The relative need of an RHA for capital is determined by the interaction of two factors: the requirements of its population for services provided through capital facilities, and the extent to which those requirements are already being met through the capital facilities currently available. In order to be able to assess relative need, therefore, it is necessary to find a way of valuing the existing capital stock.

Valuing the Stock

5.3 Valuing the capital stock entails examining both quantity and quality, since both aspects affect the amount and nature of services which can be provided and each has a direct bearing on requirements for capitalised maintenance and upgrading. No valuation method taking account of both these points was available when we started work, and we therefore set about devising one ourselves. The ideal measure of quantity and quality would no doubt be a complete survey by a single team, but experience indicates that this would be impracticable in a reasonable timescale and uneconomic. Using a number of teams would raise difficult problems of standardisation of results and although this might be overcome by appropriate statistical techniques the results might be unconvincing. We considered using energy consumption as a measure of stock capacity but this proved a poor indicator. Rateable values were also examined but after sampling tests it was found that these did not match with survey results conducted by a single team and, more importantly, were inconsistent in their mismatch. A simple bed count was considered but this did not sufficiently reflect either supporting departmental services or stock condition. All these methods were therefore rejected.

5.4 The method finally chosen was to value capital stock at its 1975 replacement cost written down to reflect its age and condition. The technique is described in detail in Annex D. Broadly, hospitals in existence at the end of 1961 were valued at 1975 bed replacement cost (including an element for back-up facilities) and written down by weighting factors appropriate to the age of each Region's stock. To this were added capital expenditure since that date and allocations for 1976/77 (also brought to a common price base and depreciated appropriately), so as to reflect renewal, upgrading and new building. Health centre accommodation was included in the valuation, but it was not possible to include other community capital stock. Account was taken of closures, downgrading and transfers of property between Regions.

5.5 This method produces an estimated valuation of RHA capital stocks, at 1975 price levels, as at the end of March 1977. It takes account both of quantity and, through the use of depreciation factors and of actual capital expenditure from 1962 onwards, of quality. It does not take account of stock which is 'wrongly' located or of a character which does not accord with policies for the delivery of service. 'Wrong' location resulting from a change in a boundary could clearly be remedied if thought necessary by redrawing boundary lines and there is no justification for spending the limited capital available on administrative tidiness of this character.

But some hospitals are badly located by any standards, and if capital were more readily available would be early candidates for replacement. However until funds are more plentiful, hospitals which are capable of delivering care (and are doing so) will have to remain in service. These hospitals have therefore been included in the measure of stock, though their mislocation could certainly be expected to influence planning in the use of resources allocated to RHAs. Similar arguments lead to the conclusion that inappropriate stock (TB sanatoria, psychiatric hospitals for example) must also continue to be counted as stock, but the valuation system should ensure that they are not highly valued. While the approach described is fairly coarse, we believe that it is about as good a relative measure of the value of capital stock and its ability to deliver care as can be obtained and is sufficiently accurate to identify significant stock deficiencies. **We recommend its adoption.**

MATCHING STOCK VALUE TO STOCK REQUIREMENTS

5.6 Once stock values have been established it is possible to set about relating them to stock requirements. The total capital wealth of the NHS consists of the value of existing stock together with new capital money available for distribution. The shares RHAs should have – their 'targets' – can be calculated by making a notional distribution of the total NHS capital wealth in proportion to their weighted populations. The system for weighting the population is similar in principle to that used for revenue purposes, but with certain necessary differences as follows:

5.6.1 *Population base.* The population base used in the proposed revenue formula is the most recent available estimate of the mid-year population of each Region. In the past for capital distribution purposes a population figure projected some 10 or 15 years ahead has been used. We consider that a 10–15 year projection can result in unnecessary investment ahead of actual population growth, and that this sort of forward look is more appropriate to planning than to construction. We should aim to provide capital to match the population nearer to the date on which the project comes into use, and consider that population projected for 5 years ahead, and rolled forward a year at a time, represents a reasonable match against planning projections, but at the same time carries little or no danger of providing unnecessary resources. We further consider that both age/sex utilisation patterns and mortality patterns are likely to remain substantially unchanged over a 5-year period, and can reasonably be applied to weight population for capital purposes.

5.6.2 *Cross-boundary patient flows.* In the proposed revenue formula we have recommended that the cost of services for people who cross Regional boundaries for in-patient treatment should be credited to the Region in which they are treated. If similar arrangements were adopted as far as capital is concerned, 'undesirable' cross-boundary flows might be perpetuated (allowance should however be made for agency and extra-territorial management arrangements). We consider therefore that inter-Regional cross-boundary flows should be disregarded in the main for capital allocation purposes although it is recognised that not all cross-boundary flows are undesirable or in a practical sense remediable. Examples are the Regional specialties and 'centres of excellence' where in the interests of efficiency some cross-boundary flows should continue for the foreseeable future. Suitable cross-accounting arrangements should be made for these outside the regular formula by agreement between the RHAs concerned. The adjustment for revenue purposes designed to compensate RHAs for the numbers of long-stay psychiatric patients who crossed boundaries before the year 1971 should not be made for capital purposes.

5.6.3 *Weighting factors.* We consider that the weighting factors recommended for the revenue formula should be applied to the capital formula except in the following respects:

5.6.3.1 *Community services.* We consider that the age weights used for revenue are not appropriate for capital since they reflect the use, in revenue expenditure terms, made of certain services (such as school health) which consume little NHS capital. We think that a better measure although not fully comprehensive is GP consultation rates (excluding telephone conversations and visits to patients' homes) by age and sex, based on 3 years' aggregated data from the General Household Survey.

5.6.3.2 *FPC Administration.* Since the expenditure involved is minimal, we recommend that a separate population base should not be taken into account.

Establishing capital targets
5.7 This process results in six separate weighted populations for each Region. We recommend that these populations should be combined to form a single weighted population for each Region based on estimated national proportional capital spending on the services concerned for the next three years. The total capital wealth of the NHS should be notionally

distributed between RHAs in proportion to population weighted as above; no allowance should be made for the London Weighting factors used in the revenue formula. Distance from target can then be assessed by comparing the target distribution with the existing stock value which has been measured in each Region. The process is described in more detail and illustrated in Annex D. We take the view that no account should be taken initially, in annual reassessments of existing stock value or of the target distribution, of transfers made by Health Authorities between revenue and capital allocations. It would however be desirable to review the capital position after a few years' operation of the system to ensure that gross new imbalances were not arising. **We recommend setting RHA capital targets by notionally distributing the total capital wealth of the NHS in proportion to population weighted as described in paragraph 5.6.**

5.8 We also considered the possibility of using population weighted in exactly the same way as for revenue for part of the capital allocation, as the revenue weights seemed more relevant for certain capital spending such as purchases of equipment and vehicles. On a 5-year population projection, however, the results would not have been significantly different from those given by using the method recommended above. We therefore decided not to pursue this possibility.

PROGRESS TOWARDS RHA CAPITAL TARGETS

5.9 Ultimately our objective is to bring about a situation in which all new capital can be distributed to RHAs on a weighted population basis. In order to do so, it will be necessary to reduce the historic disparities in the value of existing stock to an acceptable level. This should take place as quickly as is practicable, bearing in mind:

5.9.1 RHAs' capacity to absorb additional funds. Time is required first to draw up considered plans for each RHA in accordance with capital resource assumptions which may have been significantly changed, then to plan and design specific schemes and finally for construction.

5.9.2 The need to ensure that each RHA is placed in a position to meet its contractual commitments and, where appropriate, carry through consequential developments planned on the basis of earlier resource assumptions, while having sufficient 'free' capital to sustain its capital stock and promote new developments with particular regard to the needs of deprived localities.

5.9.3 The need for all RHAs to progress towards equality as smoothly as possible, so as to facilitate effective planning.

5.10 There is a level of minimum expenditure which every RHA must have in order to sustain its capital stock; and if it is to promote even modest developments by way of upgrading and developing new facilities, it needs a minimum level of capital for this purpose. Furthermore, the existing commitments of Authorities do not proportionately represent the share of capital they would receive on a 'need' basis; nevertheless, they, together with necessary consequential developments, must be met if waste is to be avoided. A transitional phase is required during which commitments can be taken into account while minimum expenditure is maintained. In order to meet these requirements, we propose that, during the period while disparities in existing stock are being ironed out, capital should be allocated on two separate bases:

5.10.1 First, a 'set minimum' level of capital should be allocated to each RHA without regard to relative shortfall in the stock: we explain in paragraphs 5.12 to 5.14 below the basis of the calculation we recommend.

5.10.2 Second, the balance of capital should be allocated to those RHAs which are shown to be short of stock in proportion to their shortfall, subject, as explained in paragraphs 5.15 and 5.16 below, to an overriding 'ceiling'.

5.11 We base our detailed recommendations on allocation of capital on the assumption that the broadly stable level of resources forecast in the White Paper, Public Expenditure to 1979/80 (Cmnd 6393), will be maintained in subsequent years. Substantial variations from year to year might make some modification of our recommendations necessary. Minor fluctuations should, we suggest, be accommodated by pro rata adjustment of RHA allocations. To illustrate the general effect of our proposals we have adopted figures suggested by the Annexes to Health Circular (76) 29, taking no account, since our purpose is solely to illustrate, of minor fluctuations and ignoring a number of factors which will affect the actual level of capital resources available to RHAs even if our assumption about the resources available nationally proves valid. Our illustration (in Annex D) thus takes no account of:

5.11.1 Future closures: these would be taken into account in the annual reassessment of stock value with consequent adjustments to the measure of shortfall from target.

5.11.2 Future disposals: these will provide RHAs with capital funds additional to their allocations; use made of these funds would be taken into account in reassessing the value of stock.

5.11.3 Transfer of resources between capital and revenue: we propose in paragraph 5.7 above that such transfers should not be taken into account year by year in assessing the value of stock but they will affect the level of capital expenditure a RHA can undertake.

The 'Floor' or 'Set Minimum'

5.12 *Short-term.* Commitments have already been entered into for forward years which must be honoured. Plans have also been set in hand on the basis of assumptions predating our analysis of existing stock values. To ensure a smooth transition **we recommend that for 1977/78 the 'set' minimum for each RHA should be 90% of the planning assumption already promulgated by the DHSS for that year, and that for 1978/79 it should be 80% of the assumption promulgated for that year.** For these two years these proportions provide a 'floor' similar to that which, for revenue, we have proposed should be set by reference to existing allocations.

5.13 *Longer-term.* Once this initial period is over there will still be a need to ensure a minimum level of capital allocation to all RHAs. **We recommend that from 1979/80 onwards the 'set minimum' achieved by allocating on a weighted population basis should be the following proportions of available capital:**

> i. **during each of the years 1979/80 to 1981/82 – 70%**
> ii. **during each of the years 1982/83 to 1984/85 – 80%**
> iii. **during each of the years 1985/86 to 1986/87 – 90%**

The balance, ie 30%, 20% and 10% respectively becomes available for distribution to RHAs falling short of their targets.

5.14 The distributional arrangements described in the foregoing paragraphs apply to all RHAs and ensure a minimum level for each RHA: for the relatively overprovided RHAs, this level remains as their maximum; for the rest it is their minimum level to be augmented by a shortfall element.

5.15 The amount allocated to each RHA for this shortfall element would be proportionate to its shortfall from target, but subject to a 'ceiling' designed to ensure that growth took place at a rate every RHA could sensibly cope with. Following informal enquiries of a number of RHAs, we suggest that this 'ceiling' level should be related to the share of total capital available each RHA could expect to receive if all the capital were distributed on the basis of weighted population. **For 1977/78 we recommend that the 'ceiling' should be set at 110% of the population-based share, rising by stages of 10% per annum until it reaches 140%, which should remain the 'ceiling' level thereafter.** This should ensure a smooth curve of growth for all RHAs as they build up their capacity. Capital released by the operation of the ceiling would be redistributed to other RHAs in a shortfall situation proportionately to their shortfall.

Smoothing the Progression

5.16 These proposals will provide a reasonably smooth progression but we believe it necessary to adopt one further constraint to ensure, in particular at the point of change-over in the basis of calculation of the 'set minimum' from existing planning assumptions to weighted population, that there can be no sudden increases or decreases from one year to the next of such a magnitude as to militate against long-term planning. **We accordingly recommend that from 1978/79 changes from one year to the next should be limited to 20% of the earlier year's allocation** (in this form our recommendation assumes stability in the level of resources available nationally: in a more generalised form it may be expressed as limiting change from one year to the next in the *percentage* of national resources received by a RHA to 20% of the earlier year's percentage).

Method of Distribution to RHAs

5.17 Annex D illustrates the effects of the proposals above. **We recommend that capital funds be distributed to RHAs in accordance with their relative positions as measured by their weighted populations and the value of existing stock in relation to their weighted populations, until such time as weighted population alone can be the criterion, subject to the operation of transitional arrangements on the lines outlined in paragraphs 5.10 to 5.16.**

Distribution of Capital below Regional Level

5.18 In the case of capital the remedying of inequalities between AHAs and Districts has to be viewed over a much longer time-scale than that appropriate to revenue. While it is possible, in revenue terms, to make a small move each year in the desired direction, the general level of capital funds likely to be available means that few large schemes can proceed simultaneously. Capital (except for minor schemes) must, therefore, be concentrated on selected projects and not so dispersed that it cannot sustain a meaningful capital programme, as would be the case if progress were attempted in every District at once. Nevertheless, the goal of equalisation should be firmly kept in view, though progress towards it will inevitably have to move in stages rather than a smooth curve.

5.19 **We recommend that RHAs should undertake a valuation of capital assets by Districts within Areas in a manner similar to that used for Regions, as described in Annex D, in order to establish relative deprivation within Regions.** The resultant 'league tables' should be used as a planning tool when deciding the allocation of new capital works – the aim would be to achieve a measure of equality over a period of years. The data for the valuation process would have to be provided locally and the population base would need to take account of those cross-boundary patient flows which RHAs consider desirable.

5.20 No such constraints apply to capital for minor schemes. While the proportion of capital money available for such schemes in each Region will vary in accordance with differences in local needs and policies, all RHAs will be distributing some capital to AHAs for such schemes, and the basis should be consistent with the principles of equity adopted nationally. **We recommend using the 'revenue' weighted population as a yardstick,** since expenditure of this nature will be related more closely to the needs of the current rather than a projected population, and the 'revenue' weighted population will already have been derived in each Region for revenue purposes. RHAs may for legitimate reasons wish to vary from the allocation indicated by the yardstick and in such cases they should make known their reasons for doing so, and discuss them with AHAs.

SPECIAL CASES

New Towns

5.21 It has been put to us that special allowance might be made for uneven distribution of New Towns between RHAs in a capital allocation formula. New Towns vary widely in planned size, rate of development and in location relative to existing services. Patients in New Towns are in no different a position from patients in many other places and we can see no justification for making an exception in their case from the rule that Regional capital requirements must be judged in relation to the needs of the projected population and the facilities available to meet those needs. In reaching this judgment we have taken note of the fact that no special allowance is made for the needs of New Towns in determining the finance to be made available for health nationally, though in other fields of public service there is a New Towns subvention. It seems to us inappropriate to depart from the practice adopted nationally when considering allocations to RHAs. Below Regional level, however, there may be special problems associated with particular New Towns, and RHAs will no doubt take these into account when judging their needs and priorities against those of other parts of the Region.

Teaching Hospitals and Health Centres

5.22 In the proposals in this chapter it has been assumed that the Department should continue to fund completely the additional capital cost of providing facilities for medical teaching, ie that special allocations covering 35 % of the total NHS cost (works, fees and equipment) of approved schemes with a total NHS cost of £350,000 or more should be made for all teaching hospital schemes. It has also been assumed that finance for health centres will continue to be included in the general RHA allocation.

CONCLUSIONS AND SUMMARY OF RECOMMENDATIONS

5.23 In this chapter we have explained the considerations which have led us to propose different criteria and methods for capital distribution from those recommended for revenue. Recognising the need to take account of the existing stock position, we have explained the practical problems of measurement and the methods whose adoption we recommend in order to overcome them. We have discussed the importance of balancing the assessment of the need of a Region's population for health service capital against the extent to which that need is already met through the existing stock; and have proposed a way of combining these elements in order to arrive at an overall assessment of each RHA's relative need for capital. As for revenue, we recognise that the pace at which imbalances can be remedied will be governed by practical considerations, and we have recommended how such considerations should be taken into account. We have also discussed the application below Regional level of the principles recommended for distribution to RHAs. The recommendations in this chapter can be summarised as follows:

5.23.1 **Existing capital stock** in each Region should be valued by the method described in Annex D (paragraphs 5.3 – 5.5).

5.23.2 **Population** should be weighted for capital purposes in a way similar to that used for revenue, with the modifications set out in Annex D (paragraphs 5.6 and 5.7).

5.23.3 **Capital targets** for RHAs should be set by notionally distributing total existing stock value and new capital money available for distribution in proportion to weighted population (paragraph 5.7).

5.23.4 **Progress towards capital targets** should take place as fast as possible, subject to the operation of special transitional arrangements in the early years (paragraph 5.12), of a 'set minimum' arrangement designed to secure a minimum share of available capital for all RHAs (paragraph 5.13) and of a 'ceiling' arrangement controlling the rate of growth to take account of practical considerations (paragraph 5.15), with safeguards against excessively rapid change (paragraph 5.16).

5.23.5 **Capital should be distributed** to RHAs in accordance with their relative positions as measured by their weighted populations and the value of existing stock in relation to their weighted populations, until such time as weighted population alone can be the criterion, subject to the arrangements referred to in paragraph 5.23.4 (paragraph 5.17).

5.23.6 **Capital assets of Districts** within Areas should be valued by RHAs in a manner similar to that described in Annex D, and the resultant 'league table' should influence the allocation of new capital works, with the aim of moving towards greater equality over time (paragraph 5.19).

5.23.7 **Capital for minor schemes** should be distributed to AHAs in accordance with population weighted as for revenue (paragraph 5.20).

CHAPTER VI   The Way Forward

THE RECOMMENDATIONS AS A WHOLE

6.1   In formulating all of our recommendations, we have borne in mind the philosophy underlying our terms of reference as set out in Chapter I. In considering methodology we have tried so far as possible to adopt a consistent approach, ie in each situation to identify relative need, to compare that need with existing provision and to suggest a practical plan for progress from existing to new patterns of allocation.

6.2   The system which we recommend for revenue allocations from the DHSS to RHAs, and for the crucial allocations to AHAs and Districts, comprises the following elements:

6.2.1   'Targets' are set for revenue allocations for services for each year at each level of allocation on the basis that the sum available nationally is apportioned successively to RHAs, AHAs and Districts in proportion to relative needs measured by population served weighted to reflect age, sex, fertility, mortality and marital status and adjusted to take account of patients crossing administrative boundaries for treatment and so far as practicable for cost differences.

6.2.2   Progress from actual allocations for the previous year towards revenue target allocations is made as fast as is consistent with practical constraints on the pace of change (expressed for purposes of RHA allocations as 'floors' and 'ceilings', and for sub-Regional allocations in a more flexible form), subject to protection from the general redistributive machinery of the additional service costs necessarily incurred as a result of training medical and dental students.

6.2.3   The service increment for medical and dental teaching is calculated for RHAs on the forecast student numbers, and below Regional level in accordance with criteria including, as a key yardstick, forecast student numbers.

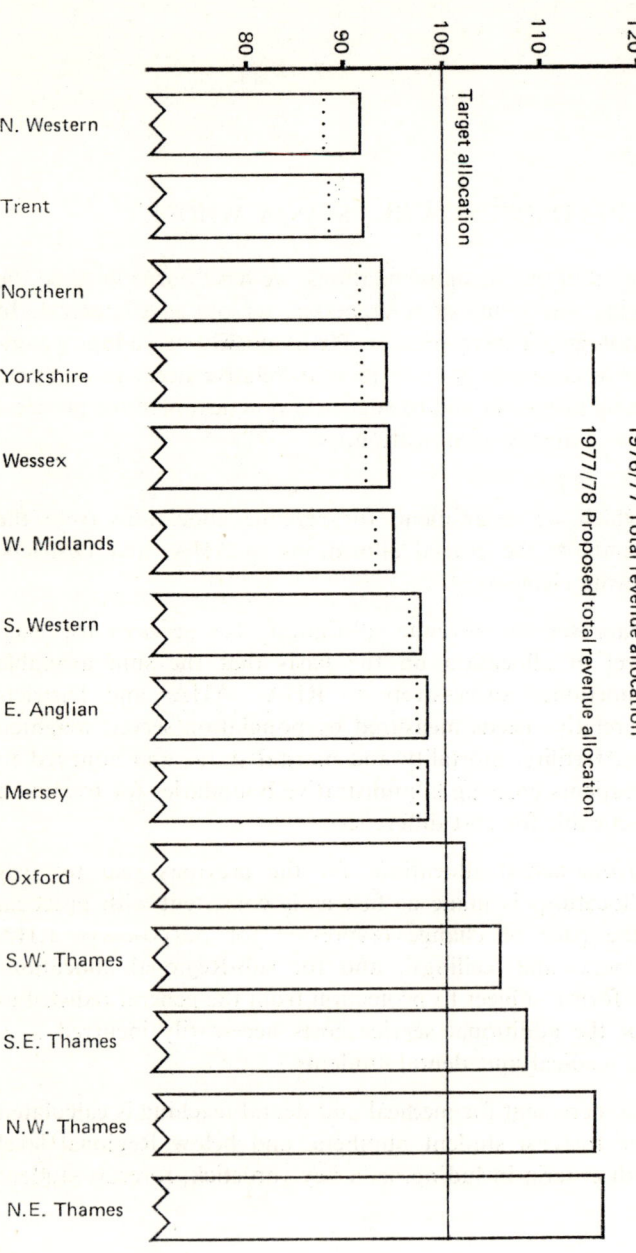

Figure VI-1   Effects of proposals on revenue allocations for 1977/78
(assuming 1.5% national growth)
Chart illustrating relationship to target
allocation in each health region

. . . . . . 1976/77 Total revenue allocation

———— 1977/78 Proposed total revenue allocation

6.3   The system we recommend for capital allocations from the DHSS to RHAs, and from RHAs to AHAs, comprises the following elements:

6.3.1   'Targets' are set each year of the share appropriate to each RHA of the combined total of the national value of capital stock (as assessed by methods devised by the Working Party) and the capital sum available for distribution; the apportionment being on the basis of population weighted largely as for revenue.

6.3.2   Progress is made from the existing value of capital stock in each RHA towards the RHA stock targets as fast as is consistent with the capital funds available each year, the commitments for existing capital work and practical constraints on the pace of change expressed as 'set minima' and 'ceilings'.

6.3.3   Capital devoted by RHAs to Areas for minor capital works should have regard, as a yardstick, to the weighted populations of the Areas as used for the revenue allocation process.

6.3.4   Capital allocations from RHAs to AHAs for other capital works should have regard, as a yardstick, to stock values in the Areas measured in a way similar to that used for the Region as a whole.

EFFECTS OF THE CHANGES RECOMMENDED

Revenue

6.4   Significant improvements are suggested in the criteria of need to be used in future, compared with those on which allocations were based for 1976/77 following our first Interim Report. Our original appraisal of the relative needs of RHAs can now be reviewed in the light of the more sensitive measures developed, and a number of changes are revealed in the targets towards which each should be moving, though changes in actual allocations in any one year would of course be considerably less marked due to the operation of 'floors' and 'ceilings'. Figure VI-1 illustrates the effects our proposals would have on revenue allocations in 1977/78, subject to certain assumptions.

6.5   Figure VI-2 shows the effect, in terms of the percentage swing of each RHA in relation to its revenue target, when the 1976/77 position is compared with 1977/78 with the recommended changes applied as fully as the data permit at this stage. A $1\frac{1}{2}\%$ growth nationally has been assumed for 1977/78. The largest swings are seen to take place in the North Western, Trent, Northern, Mersey, North West Thames and North East Thames RHAs, whilst Wessex, South Western, East Anglian, South West Thames and South East Thames are affected very much less.

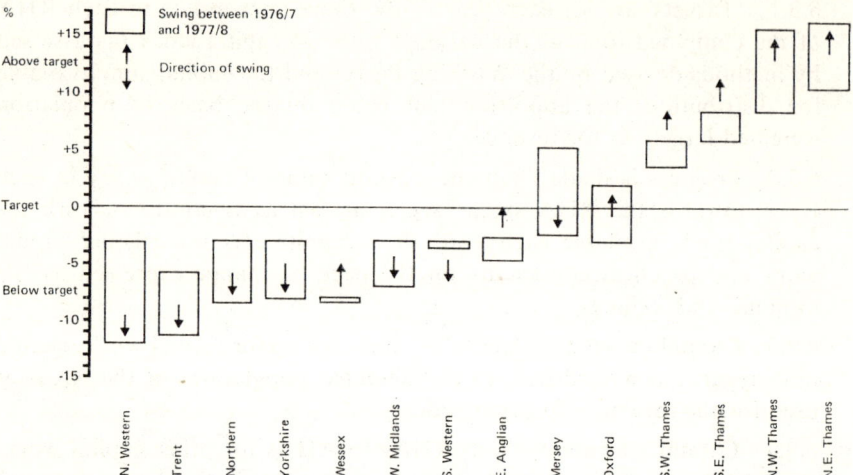

Figure VI-2 Swings between 1976/77 and 1977/78

6.6　The swings illustrated in Figure VI-2 are the net result of individual changes which are not only different in magnitude in each RHA, but which may also pull in different directions. The swings are analysed by component elements in Figure VI-3:

Figure VI-3 Analysis of swings in figure VI-2

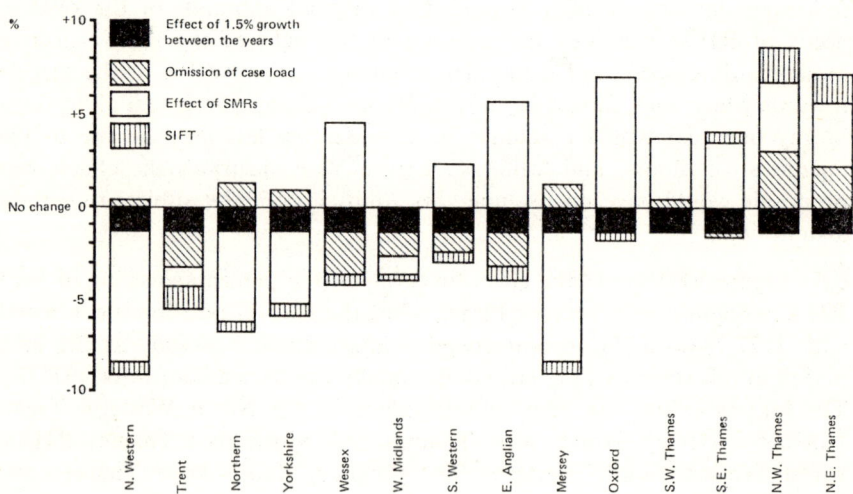

6.7   The change having the greatest effect is the introduction of a morbidity factor based upon SMRs. This was predictable and affects North Western, East Anglian, Mersey and Oxford more than others. The formula combines expected bed utilisation and SMRs by condition and the results are therefore influenced largely by those conditions having a high bed usage. North Western and Mersey, for example, both have above average SMRs for most conditions, the highest SMRs in each case being for conditions which take up about one-third of the country's general hospital beds. Both have high SMRs – in North Western's case the highest – for cardiovascular diseases which take up about one-quarter of all general hospital beds. By contrast East Anglian and Oxford have below average SMRs for most conditions and particularly for those which have a high bed usage.

6.8   Elimination of the caseload factor, which as we have already mentioned is supply-dominated, has a differential effect, quantitatively, broadly in proportion to the relationship between caseload and the weighted population in each Region. The direction of the swing will be determined by that relationship. Thus in Regions which tend to have too few beds in relation to their population, the effect of eliminating the caseload factor is to push them further below or down towards their target and vice versa. The relationship is not quite as simple as this since relative efficiency, ie throughput of patients per bed, also plays a part.

6.9   The effect of the new approach to assessing the additional service costs arising from clinical teaching is largely to increase the apparent needs of provincial RHAs by contrast with those of the Thames RHAs. This is due primarily, as explained in Chapter IV, to the abandonment of the different levels of 'teaching and research allowance' for London and the provinces proposed in our Interim Report, which had the effect of including costs which should properly have been attributed to service needs in London, while at the same time taking insufficient account of the effects of service deprivation outside London. The adoption of a common basis for determining SIFT provides a consistent relationship between service and teaching requirements proportionate to the scale of teaching activity. As a result, however, of taking student growth into account for a further two years, the SIFT requirements of those RHAs with new and expanding medical schools are greater. The protection of larger or smaller sums in total allocations affects the distance from target and establishes a different order of relative deprivation or better provision.

Capital

6.10 Similar comparisons cannot be made for capital, since no target allocations were proposed in our Interim Report. The basis of distribution for 1976/77 was distorted by the overriding need to fund contractual commitments and the element in allocations which was based on weighted population was comparatively small. Our proposed assessment of need departs in two important respects from previous practice and to that extent from expectations based on history. First, the population weighting system differs from that previously used in the same way as for revenue, and with similar effects. Second, we are introducing for the first time a need measure based on capital stock valuation, the effect of which is to restrict for a period the level of capital investment in East Anglian, North West Thames, North East Thames, South West Thames, Oxford and Mersey in favour of the remaining RHAs. Unless such an adjustment is made, distribution by reference to weighted population as the sole criterion would tend to perpetuate indefinitely the historic differences in the availability and condition of capital stock in a way incompatible with the objectives underlying the proposed revenue distribution arrangements.

BALANCE BETWEEN CAPITAL AND REVENUE

6.11 In the opening chapter of this Report, we drew attention to the importance of establishing the right balance between capital and revenue expenditure. Although based on similar principles, the distributional methods recommended for each kind of expenditure have different characteristics. This is inevitable so long as the geographical disparities in quantity and quality of capital stock remain. The equalisation process we recommend for capital distribution is based upon capital stock valuation. We must emphasise, however, that the equalisation it produces is a relative equalisation only and does not in itself necessarily achieve the right quantum of capital stock in each geographic location. The method is necessary as a means of distributing the available new capital in the fairest possible way but, because of the limited amount of capital which can be made available annually, providing an adequate capital stock in every locality may take a long time to achieve.

6.12 Many real problems remain. Deprived RHAs who can expect to enjoy a relatively higher growth rate in their revenue allocations will inevitably be forced to invest capital in buildings and facilities. Their capacity to do so will be seriously restricted if they rely solely on the finance distributed as capital. Indeed unless this can be augmented there is a real risk that rising revenue expenditure will not be absorbed in an economic way. Correspondingly, RHAs whose revenue growth is likely to be severely restricted may also have an excess of capital stock, although much of it may be valued at a lower level and also be mislocated. These RHAs may also need to invest in capital development at least in the short term if they are to secure a more effective and economical distribution of their resources. The permutations between capital stock and revenue deployment are almost infinitely variable, both between and within Regions.

6.13   Consideration of these problems leads naturally to the proposition that an arbitrary distinction between capital and revenue expenditure is undesirable. If the distinction could be eliminated, Authorities would be free to pursue capital investment policies which were designed to achieve a balance between capital and revenue expenditure judged most appropria e to the local situation. As well as practical difficulties there are objections of principle to this approach. Overall control of the level of investment of public expenditure in capital enterprises is essential to the national economy to avoid damaging effects on the construction industry, to maintain the best balance between public and private investment and to secure the most economic utilisation of national resources.

6.14   There are ways in which the difficulties can be overcome. The essential nature of the problem has already been recognised in the increased flexibility between capital and revenue expenditure introduced in 1975/76 and extended in 1976/77. These arrangements allow Authorities, at their discretion, to transfer to capital account up to 1% of their revenue allocation or up to 10% of their capital allocation to revenue. This greater freedom is very much welcomed and will go a long way towards enabling RHAs to overcome the shortages of capital stock to which we have referred above and to secure a better balance between investment and consumption. It has been represented to us, however, that the permitted limits of transfer-ability are still too restrictive for a RHA which needed to achieve a major strategic realignment of its services and required therefore to embark on a higher level of capital investment. Nor does the restriction allow much scope for capital-based developments aimed at securing an eventual reduction in running costs.

6.15   For the above reasons we consider it essential – and are advised that it is practicable – to allow RHAs to seek an augmentation of their future capital allocations at the expense of their future revenue allocations and vice versa over and above the permitted limit of flexibility within the year. The revenue and capital allocations for the years in question would be adjusted within the same overall total. To preserve the equalisation effects of the revenue distributional formula the revenue and capital allocations for the forward year(s) would first be calculated disregarding such adjustments; the adjustment would be made afterwards in the notified allocation forecasts. The forecasts would enable the Department to arrange a national capital/revenue apportionment in the forward years which reflected as far as possible the planning intentions of the Authorities. Actual expenditure would continue to be brought to account as revenue or capital as the case may be and strictly in accordance with the definition of capital expenditure.

6.16 The arrangement described above would permit much greater flexibility in strategic planning and give Authorities more room to manoeuvre while at the same time retaining the tactical freedom conferred by the existing flexibility limits. **We therefore recommend that RHAs should be allowed to seek an augmentation of their future capital allocations at the expense of their future revenue allocations and vice versa over and above the permitted level of flexibility within the year.**

6.17 In the course of our deliberations on this issue, we examined other alternatives. One method of achieving much the same objective, the 'bidding' approach, is described in Annex E. We rejected it as being too complex for present use and because it might potentially create some uncertainty in long term plans. But because it has some intrinsic merits we think it useful to record – others may consider it worthwhile exploring further at a future date.

EXPENDITURE ON FAMILY PRACTITIONER SERVICES

6.18 Our terms of reference limit our consideration to the resources allocated to Health Authorities and therefore to the needs of populations for the services which those Authorities themselves provide. These include the administrative expenses of the Family Practitioner Committees, which are provided for in Health Authority allocations. Resources made available to Health Authorities for the provision of family practitioner services are provided in an entirely different way and to an extent are open-ended.

6.19 But there can be no doubt that many of the services provided by family practitioners have an important impact on those provided by the Health Authorities and vice versa. It is also self-evident that they should both respond, each in their own way, to the same criteria of need. Such evidence as is available to us suggests that there are significant geographical disparities in the levels of provision of family practitioner services just as there are, for example, in the hospital services. Subjectively, we would consider it surprising if these disparities turned out to be compensatory or if one was the cause or effect of the other. In terms of total expenditure the degree of financial overlap may be small but, in terms of resource restriction affecting the Health Authority controlled services, even minor overlaps may considerably influence decisions as to how services should be provided at the margins.

6.20 It is, to say the least, credible that the effect of the separate funding arrangements and the lack of a common need base may well lead to diverse and possibly incompatible planning decisions. In general, direct aid from Health Authorities to strengthen primary care is to be welcomed, since national policy seeks to achieve a shift of resources from secondary to primary care services. In other cases the way in which primary care is delivered may actually contribute to the load to be borne by the secondary care services.

6.21 Whilst we recognise fully the many difficult issues involved, we consider that if the objective underlying our terms of reference is to be fulfilled, ways need to be found of securing that the resources at present allocated in quite different ways are more closely related so that the impact of geographical disparities in one part of the service or another is taken into account. One way of so doing might be to take account where appropriate of geographic FPS expenditure in determining allocations to Health Authorities. We suggest that a review of the interaction between the two services from a financial viewpoint would be timely and **we recommend that it should be undertaken.**

INFORMATION AND RESEARCH NEEDS

6.22 We believe our recommendations to be the best possible, given the data currently available. We are in no doubt that the measures we have used are adequate to establish the right direction for change and can stand for some years to come. At the same time we see a clear and pressing need for improvement in the data routinely collected and for achieving through research a better appreciation and understanding of the factors on which future resource allocation decisions need to be based. It is, in our view, unlikely that such improvements would call into question any of the principles established in this Report. They would, however, provide an improved basis for their application and would enable need to be measured with greater confidence and sensitivity as disparities are reduced to a level at which roughnesses which are tolerable at present begin to assume greater importance.

Routine Data Collection

6.23 A mass of information is collected regularly about NHS activities and facilities. Much of this is difficult to use to the full for allocation purposes because of problems in linking statistics from different data sources. Furthermore, despite the scale of the operation, important gaps still exist. Outpatients represent almost as large a proportion of NHS expenditure as all psychiatric patients, yet virtually nothing is known about their characteristics and movements. Community care, including family practitioner services, is a significant and increasing element in NHS provision, yet the data collected on these services fall far short in comprehensiveness and reliability of those on hospital in-patients.

6.24 We are aware that the system for collecting costing information is still in the process of development. There is a long way to go before the costs of the component activities of the NHS can be comprehensively analysed with absolute confidence in the result. Existing methods of assessing specialty costs are open to improvement; costs relating to specific conditions have yet to be established. Examination is needed of the differences in NHS costs for the same level of service in different localities, whether due to market factors or to differences in modes of delivery of service, including the impact of family practitioner services on other aspects of health care. Better means are needed of distinguishing between service and teaching costs, and identifying the nature and desirability of costs arising from 'excellence' – though this last point impinges on the difficult field of outcome measures, where work is still in its very early stages.

6.25 **We recommend that data requirements be kept under review, both with regard to the identification and elimination of information gaps and with a view to ensuring compatibility of data from different sources so as to facilitate linkage and analysis.**

Fundamental Research

6.26 Data collection is useless unless it is guided by a clear understanding of the uses for which the information is required. In the context of resource allocation the key problem is measurement of need for health services and the key areas for research are:

6.26.1 Validation of those criteria currently used or available.

6.26.2 The search for new criteria to supplement or replace those currently used. Evidence we have received suggests that a number of sources of information exist which might yield improvements in the sensitivity of need criteria for particular services on detailed exploration.

We recommend the setting up of a group of Departmental officials and expert advisers drawn from outside the Department to consider how research might best proceed. We are able to make available to such a group all the evidence received offering suggestions for research which we have been unable to pursue.

Priorities

6.27 In exposing the deficiencies in the knowledge which exists, we are conscious of the need to draw a clear distinction between what it is essential to know in order to have a reliable and acceptable basis for resource allocation and what is necessary to promote a better understanding of resource utilisation. Collecting and processing information is expensive and time-consuming for all concerned. In a time of economic restraint, it would be difficult to argue that a very high priority should automatically be accorded to the gathering of new information relative to resource allocation unless it can be shown to be likely to have a material and significant effect on the process.

6.28 Research is a rather different matter and its benefits are likely to be longer rather than shorter term and to have implications wider than the narrow issue of resource allocation. We believe it important for research to be mounted in the areas indicated and that it should be accorded a reasonably high priority. **We recommend accordingly.**

SUMMARY OF RECOMMENDATIONS

6.29 The recommendations in this chapter can be summarised as follows:

6.29.1 **New arrangements for flexibility** between capital and revenue should be introduced in addition to the retention of the existing arrangements (paragraphs 6.14–6.16).

6.29.2 **A review of the interaction** between FPS expenditure and all other health expenditure should be undertaken (paragraph 6.21).

6.29.3 **Data requirements** should be kept under review (paragraph 6.25).

6.29.4 **Research requirements** should be considered by a group of Departmental officials and expert advisers from outside the Department and should command reasonable priority (paragraphs 6.26 and 6.28).

CONCLUSIONS

6.30 As we said at the beginning of this Report, the proposals which we have put forward are final only in the sense that we believe we have taken the study as far as it can possibly be taken within the limitations of the data available and the interpretation which may be placed upon them. Our conclusions are unanimous. We firmly believe them to be valid and relevant to the needs of the NHS as a whole, and that they should be used as a basis for allocating resources for some years to come. At the same time we are very conscious of the need for further study and research, particularly in the improvement of data bases. We have identified some areas where we consider such research likely to prove beneficial by enabling the methods we have proposed to be operated with greater sensitivity. It will also, we hope, serve to promote a fuller understanding of the nature of the problem. We think it unlikely that it would call into question, in a fundamental way, the principles on which our recommendations are based or the methodology proposed for their implementation.

Morbidity

6.31 Among the changes recommended, that which has the greatest effect is the use of SMRs to take account of the known geographical variations in morbidity. Our purpose has been to ensure that resources are made available to enable Health Authorities to meet the needs which arise from the morbidity of the populations which they serve. We recognise that the prevalence of many of the conditions which are among the main causes of mortality is probably not significantly influenced by the intervention of health care services and that the redistribution of resources may not therefore have a significant and early impact on morbidity characteristics. But this cannot be a reason for ignoring them, since the NHS has a statutory responsibility to respond to the needs which those characteristics generate.

6.32 Marginal though the impact of health care services delivered after the event may be on morbidity patterns, mortality and morbidity can be significantly influenced by positive preventive measures (eg by promoting changes in smoking habits) and by encouraging improvements in the environment in which people live and work (eg better housing and working conditions). The necessity to promote preventive measures is countrywide, but the need is almost certainly greater where the mortality ratios are high. Health Authorities have a leading, though not an exclusive, responsibility in this field.

6.33 For both the above reasons, therefore, we are convinced that it is essential to recognise morbidity variations in resource allocation and the method we have proposed does so in the best way possible in present circumstances.

Relationship to Planning

6.34 Whilst, as we have said earlier, resource allocation is not directly concerned with the way in which resources are actually deployed, it has of course a very considerable influence on the planning process. The methods we propose for determining allocations will also provide a critical tool in planning by providing a need-related baseline showing the share of the available resource which should be consumed by a given population. The formulation of resource targets is clearly an important first step in planning the provision of services. If what we propose is accepted, some localities will gain, some will be constrained, while others will suffer a reduction in resource currently available. The inevitable consequences of introducing a fairer method of distribution of resources are likely to gain widespread public support only if they are seen to influence the actual provision of services in the way intended. For this reason we draw particular attention to the importance of following through our proposals effectively in the planning process which will make their impact explicit.

Practical Consequences

6.35 We have tried to keep our proposals as straightforward as possible, but some complexity is unavoidable. We have also constantly borne in mind the work entailed in implementing them. We are certain that they are practicable but we are also very conscious of the considerable initial task of assembling the data necessary to operate them, calculating the targets and determining and consulting on actual allocations particularly at the sub-Regional level. This task will fall heavily on NHS management staff at a time when they are being asked to economise in their management costs. We cannot estimate precisely what will be involved but we are sure that in the first year or so the effort required will be significant at all levels. We urge strongly, therefore, that this should be fully recognised when decisions are reached on the current review of management costs.

The Future of the Working Party
6.36 We have discharged the main task laid upon us by our terms of reference. There remain, however, some important aspects requiring further study which ought not to be delayed, notably the impact of market conditions on the costs of providing services and the relationship between Health Authority expenditure and that of the family practitioner services. A mechanism will also be needed to consider, in due course, the results of the research we have also suggested. Whilst it would be inappropriate for us to suggest our own survival, we believe that consideration should be given to the establishment of a similarly constituted group to which resource allocation issues could be remitted as they arise.

METHODS OF WORK AND MEMBERSHIP

A1. The Working Party established sub-groups to study three aspects of its remit in detail: revenue allocations, capital allocations and the additional NHS revenue service costs necessarily associated with clinical teaching. The establishment of sub-groups enabled the Working Party to proceed more quickly and, through co-option, to widen the range of expertise at its disposal.

A2. The Working Party also sought evidence and took views and advice from various experts, in particular, on the most appropriate indicators of need for psychiatric services. It sought evidence from RHAs on the work being done towards the end of 1975 on allocations to AHAs, and studied reports of meetings held with representatives of RHAs to discuss in more detail the methodology for allocations to AHAs particularly in relation to data problems.

A3. Membership of the Working Party and its sub-groups including co-opted members is set out on the following pages.

RESOURCE ALLOCATION WORKING PARTY

LIST OF MEMBERS

Chairman: J C C Smith — Under Secretary, Regional Planning Division

NHS Members

G C Bateson — Area Administrator, Liverpool AHA (T)

Mrs P M Boulton — District Nursing Officer, South West Surrey District, Surrey AHA

I A Donaldson — District Administrator, North Teesside District, Cleveland AHA

M Fairey — Regional Administrator, North East Thames RHA

Dr J M Forsythe — Area Medical Officer, Kent AHA

Miss B Hall — Regional Nursing Officer, West Midlands RHA

Professor W W Holland — Professor of Clinical Epidemiology and Social Medicine, St Thomas' Hospital Medical School

F S Jackson — District Finance Officer, North East District (T), Kensington, Chelsea and Westminster AHA (T)

Dr A J Lane — Regional Medical Officer, North Western RHA

T Rippington — Regional Treasurer, South Western RHA

M Sharples — Area Treasurer, Tameside AHA

D Thompson — Regional Works Officer, Trent RHA

DHSS Members

Dr D Burbridge (until October 1975) — Senior Principal Medical Officer, Medical Division

B E Drake — Chief Surveyor, Surveying Division

P Fletcher — Assistant Secretary, Central Planning Division

C Graham — Assistant Secretary, Regional Planning Division

R S King (from February 1976) — Assistant Secretary, Regional Planning Division

Miss C Lester — Principal Nursing Officer, Nursing Division

J D Pole	– Senior Economic Adviser, Economic Advisers' Office
J Rowntree	– Chief Statistician, Statistics and Research Division
Dr E Shore (from February 1976)	– Senior Principal Medical Officer, Medical Division
C G Taylor	– Assistant Secretary, Finance Division
Dr C E R Tristem	– Senior Principal Scientific Officer, Operational Research Services

Secretariat

Mrs E A Woods
Miss C Baines
M E Lally
Miss S Novit

– Regional Planning Division

RESOURCE ALLOCATION WORKING PARTY – REVENUE SUB-GROUP

LIST OF MEMBERS

Chairman: C Graham	– Assistant Secretary, Regional Planning Division

NHS Members

G C Bateson	– Area Administrator, Liverpool AHA (T)
Professor A E Bennett	– Director, Department of Clinical Epidemiology, St George's Hospital
Mrs P M Boulton	– District Nursing Officer, South West Surrey District, Surrey AHA
B G Bush	– Regional Treasurer, East Anglian RHA
I A Donaldson	– District Administrator, North Teesside District, Cleveland AHA
M Fairey	– Regional Administrator, North East Thames RHA
Dr J M Forsythe	– Area Medical Officer, Kent AHA
Professor W W Holland	– Professor of Clinical Epidemiology and Social Medicine, St Thomas' Hospital Medical School
Dr A J Lane	– Regional Medical Officer, North Western RHA
M Sharples	– Area Treasurer, Tameside AHA

DHSS Members

Dr N P Halliday (from January 1976)	– Senior Medical Officer, Medical Division
Dr A B Harrington (until October 1975)	– Senior Principal Medical Officer, Medical Division
C Himatsingani	– Principal Scientific Officer, Operational Research Services
Dr A Fenton Lewis	– Senior Medical Officer, Medical Division
R C Longfield	– Principal, Regional Planning Division
J H Rickard	– Economic Adviser, Economic Advisers' Office
J Rowntree (from December 1975)	– Chief Statistician, Statistics and Research Division
M Sharratt (until October 1975)	– Statistician, Statistics and Research Division
Mrs E A Woods	– Principal, Regional Planning Division
C G Taylor	– Assistant Secretary, Finance Division
Miss S P C Wright-Warren	– Nursing Officer, Nursing Division

Secretariat

M E Lally ⎫
Miss S Novit ⎭   – Regional Planning Division

RESOURCE ALLOCATION WORKING PARTY – CAPITAL SUB-GROUP

LIST OF MEMBERS

Chairman: B E Drake	– Chief Surveyor, Surveying Division

NHS Members

A B Baker (from February 1976)	– Regional Administrator, Northern RHA
Dr J M Forsythe	– Area Medical Officer, Kent AHA
J A Hill	– Area Works Officer, Kensington, Chelsea and Westminster AHA (T)
F Pethybridge (until January 1976)	– Regional Administrator, North Western RHA
T Rippington	– Regional Treasurer, South Western RHA
D Thompson	– Regional Works Officer, Trent RHA
Miss M Walton	– Area Nursing Officer, Leeds AHA (T)

DHSS Members

Dr N P Halliday (from January 1976)	– Senior Medical Officer, Medical Division
C Himatsingani (from September 1975)	– Principal Scientific Officer, Operational Research Services
K Hudson	– Superintending Quantity Surveyor, Surveying Division
R C C Langham	– Principal, Regional Planning Division
P Mancini	– Senior Economic Assistant, Economic Advisers' Office
J H Rickard (until May 1976)	– Economic Adviser, Economic Advisers' Office
W G Robertson (until July 1975)	– Principal Scientific Officer, Operational Research Services
Mrs E A Woods	– Principal, Regional Planning Division
Dr T K Sweeney (until December 1975)	– Senior Medical Officer, Medical Division

Secretariat

D H Pepper ⎫
A Miley ⎬ – Health Building Division

RESOURCE ALLOCATION WORKING PARTY – TEACHING AND RESEARCH SUB-GROUP

LIST OF MEMBERS

Chairman: P Fletcher	– Assistant Secretary, Central Planning Division

NHS Members

M Fairey	– Regional Administrator, North East Thames RHA
Miss B Hall	– Regional Nursing Officer, West Midlands RHA
Professor W W Holland	– Professor of Clinical Epidemiology and Social Medicine, St Thomas' Hospital Medical School
B E Hulse	– Area Treasurer, Oxford AHA (T)
F S Jackson	– District Finance Officer, North East District (T), Kensington, Chelsea and Westminster AHA (T)

| M S Rigden | – Regional Treasurer, Trent RHA |
| Dr A H Snaith | – Area Medical Officer, Avon AHA (T) |

DHSS Members

D Brereton	– Principal, Central Planning Division
P W Day	– Senior Principal, Finance Division
J Hurst	– Economic Adviser, Economic Advisers' Office
R C Longfield	– Principal, Regional Planning Division
Dr J L D Radcliffe (from January 1976)	– Senior Medical Officer, Medical Division
A B Rees (until January 1976)	– Senior Principal, Regional Planning Division
Dr G R M Sichel (until September 1975)	– Senior Medical Officer, Medical Division
Mrs E A Woods	– Principal, Regional Planning Division

UGC Member
Professor Sir Charles Stuart-Harris
(from January 1976)

Secretariat
H A Jones
B J Harrison   }   – Central Planning Division
Miss V Lewis

FIRST INTERIM REPORT: AUGUST 1975

INTRODUCTION

B1. The Working Party was asked to give early consideration to recommending any improvement which could be incorporated in the methods of allocating resources to RHAs in 1976/77. The timetable offered little scope for in-depth analysis and research. The Working Party therefore limited itself, on revenue, to an examination of how best the methods used in previous years for distribution to Regions could be improved, whether the weighting factors could be modified and how far it was possible to speed up the process of equalisation in 1976/77. The Working Party similarly considered whether any improvements could be made for 1976/77 in the distribution of capital.

SUMMARY OF RECOMMENDATIONS

B2. The main recommendations were:

Revenue
B2.1 'Target' allocations, using a modified formula should be established for each RHA.

B2.2 The formula for calculating target allocations for RHAs for general service requirements, ie the funds which each RHA should receive if the total available for general services were to be allocated according to the criteria in the formula, should be based on:

B2.2.1 The national utilisation of different services by age and sex groups (cost weighted wherever possible) applied to the population structure to produce weighted populations, and

B2.2.2 A caseload factor for the hospital services reflecting the actual cases, both in- and out-patients, in each Region.

These two factors should be combined in the ratio of 3:1. Community services would be assessed on the basis of weighted population alone. The beds element in- the previous formula should be abandoned.

B2.3 RHAs should receive funds to cover the revenue consequences arising in 1976/77 from new major capital schemes.

B2.4 An allowance should be protected within the total revenue allocation to cover the additional costs of providing services as a result of the clinical teaching of medical and dental undergraduate students. In the Thames Regions this allowance should be based upon 75% of the excess cost of London Teaching Hospitals, and in other Regions upon 75% of the excess cost of Provincial Teaching Hospitals over corresponding non-teaching hospitals. The allowance should take account of the number of undergraduate students expected to be undergoing clinical training in teaching and non-teaching hospitals two years later ie in 1978/79.

B2.5 As an exceptional case, the excess costs of the Hammersmith and Northwick Park Hospitals should be protected on a similar basis as for undergraduate teaching and research, ie at a level of 75%.

B2.6 Actual allocations to RHAs should be determined according to each RHA's position in relation to its 'target allocation' subject to the operation of a 'floor' and 'ceiling' set to ensure that no RHA's final allocation decreased or increased beyond a reasonable level.

B2.7 Application of the formula should not allow any RHA to worsen its position in relation to its target ie a deprived RHA to become more deprived or a well provided RHA to become better provided.

Capital
B2.8 Capital should be distributed by reference to commitments and 1986 weighted population.

B2.9 A sum of about £8m should be distributed to certain RHAs as an interim arrangement to make a modest start towards remedying relative health deprivation through increased capital investment.

RESPONSES TO RECOMMENDATIONS AS A RESULT OF
CONSULTATIONS

B3. Interested bodies including Regional Health Authorities, professional organisations, the University Grants Committee and Committee of Vice-Chancellors and Principals, and the Staff Side of the General Whitley Council were consulted on these recommendations. The outcome showed that there was widespread and general support for the policy of distribution on the basis of relative need, and for the principles underlying the proposed revenue formula, including the concept of a teaching and research allowance, and the proposed method of distributing capital. The reservations which were expressed centred mainly on the pace at which movement towards a more equitable distribution could be achieved in 1976/77, the treatment of London compared with the provinces in the proposed teaching allowance, and that part of the teaching allowance that related to dental students, and on the proposed distribution of £8m capital for relative health deprivation. Many of those commenting also supported the Working Party's expressed intention to study additional possible criteria of need, while accepting that in the time available it was impracticable to take these into account for 1976/77.

APPLICATION TO ALLOCATIONS FOR 1976/77

B4.   On 18 February 1976 the Secretary of State in a letter to the Chairmen of Regional Health Authorities announced the decisions on the financial allocations to RHAs for 1976/77. These decisions based on the recommendations of the Working Party were as follows:

B4.1   The revenue formula used for calculating revenue targets for RHAs was to be based on the criteria recommended by the Working Party.

B4.2   The Secretary of State decided that *actual* revenue allocations were to be brought as close as was practicable and possible to target allocations for 1976/77. The result was a major step in the direction of increasing the level of resources to relatively deprived RHAs.

B4.3   All RHAs were to receive revenue funds to cover the commitments arising from their new major capital schemes.

B4.4   A floor was to be set at 0% which meant that Mersey and the four Thames RHAs received no additional funds beyond those at B4.3 but did not have to sustain any reductions.

B4.5   A ceiling was to be set at 4% which was higher than the $2\frac{1}{2}\%$ illustrated by the Working Party; this was made possible largely by an increase in the permitted flexibility between revenue and capital.

B4.6 Each RHA should have protected within its allocation a teaching allowance in the form recommended.

B4.7 Capital funds were to be allocated in line with the Working Party's recommendations except that no additional funds were to be set aside specifically for allocation to health deprived RHAs.

B4.8 The Department issued interim guidance to Authorities based on the advice of the Working Party on the distribution of financial resources to AHAs and Districts. The guidance stressed the need that as far as practicable sub-Regional allocations should be made in accordance with the principles determining RHA allocations.

DISTRIBUTION OF REVENUE FUNDS TO REGIONAL HEALTH AUTHORITIES: WEIGHTING THE POPULATION TO PRODUCE REVENUE TARGETS

C1. This annex illustrates and describes how the recommendations of the Working Party for weighting and adjusting the population bases can be implemented and how the weighting factors are derived. It discusses for each population base the weights to be used, displays the data which assisted the Working Party to make these recommendations and shows the effects of each on the population of each Region. The main features of the weighting system are dealt with in the same order as discussed in the Report.

POPULATION BASE

C2. The Report recommends using mid-year estimates of the population for each Region nearest to the year for which allocations are being made. For 1977/78, this would probably mean using 1975 mid-year estimates since 1976 estimates in the detail required are unlikely to be available in time. For the illustrative figures on revenue in this Report, 1975 mid-year estimates have been taken although for the derivation of the weights themselves the population year used has been that for which the most recent utilisation data were available.

MEASURING NEED FOR NON-PSYCHIATRIC IN-PATIENT SERVICES

C3. *Age and sex weighting factors.* The following table illustrates how the demands imposed by the different age groups for each sex on the hospital in-patient services vary:

Table C1   **NATIONAL HOSPITAL IN-PATIENT UTILISATION RATES**
by age group for each sex
in terms of non-psychiatric bed-days per 1,000 population

Age groups	Males	Females
0– 4	958	726
5–14	420	318
15–19	405	990
20–24	443	1,616
25–34	480	1,428
35–44	607	939
45–64	1,406	1,170
65–74	3,284	3,000
75+	8,191	9,805

Sources: Population – 1972 mid-year estimates; bed-days from 1972 HIPE.

C4. In order to weight the population, the national rates need to be combined with each Region's population structure. The method is to apply the above utilisation rates to each Region's 1975 population breakdown in the corresponding age/sex bands; the results are summed for each Region, thus producing in effect for each Region its expected notional share of the total national bed-days. The population of England is then apportioned to each Region in the ratio of expected Regional bed-days to national bed-days. The following table illustrates the result:

Table C2 COMPARISON BY REGION OF POPULATIONS

Crude, and weighted by age/sex non-psychiatric in-patient utilisation rates

Region	Crude population 000s	Expected bed-days	Weighted population 000s	Ratio of age/sex weighted population to crude
Northern	3,126.1	4,568,595	3,021.0	0.97
Yorkshire	3,576.9	5,429,226	3,590.1	1.00
Trent	4,545.4	6,676,110	4,414.6	0.97
East Anglian	1,780.4	2,773,292	1,833.8	1.03
NW Thames	3,475.3	5,079,591	3,358.9	0.97
NE Thames	3,717.7	5,655,839	3,739.9	1.00
SE Thames	3,603.2	5,932,994	3,923.2	1.09
SW Thames	2,880.3	4,639,339	3,067.8	1.06
Wessex	2,644.9	4,150,188	2,744.3	1.04
Oxford	2,199.3	3,084,718	2,039.8	0.93
South Western	3,148.7	5,192,738	3,433.7	1.09
West Midlands	5,178.1	7,271,325	4,808.2	0.93
Mersey	2,499.3	3,612,165	2,388.5	0.96
North Western	4,078.1	6,185,057	4,089.9	1.00
England	46,453.7	70,251,177	46,453.7	1.00

Sources: Population – 1975 mid-year estimates; weighting factors from Table C1.

C5. *Standardised Mortality Ratios.* The charts and maps reproduced in Chapter II illustrate graphically the variations in overall SMRs in different parts of the country. The following table shows for males and females the SMRs for each Regional Hospital Board area in 1971 but for convenience they are displayed by reference to Regional Health Authority; more recent data on a RHA basis were not available at the time these illustrations were prepared:

Table C3   STANDARDISED MORTALITY RATIOS BY
REGION

Region	Males	Females
Northern	110	107
Yorkshire	106	104
Trent	101	102
East Anglian	88	92
NW Thames	94	97
NE Thames	97	95
SE Thames	93	96
SW Thames	94	96
Wessex	89	91
Oxford	88	91
South Western	94	96
West Midlands	103	101
Mersey	113	110
North Western	112	109

Sources: Population – 1971 mid-year estimates; SMRs for 1971.

C6. The SMRs for each Region should be linked to the age/sex weighting in such a way that the weighted population produced for each Region by the age/sex utilisation rates as above is adjusted by reference to the appropriate SMR's value. Thus a SMR value of 1.05 would result in a 5% increase in the weighted population calculated for that Region by reference to age/sex utilisation rates. A more sensitive method of applying SMRs for the non-psychiatric in-patient services is obtained by disaggregating the SMRs and the age/sex utilisation rates into the following broad groups of conditions. Weight can then be given to the differential bed utilisation rates associated with each condition. The groups of conditions are based upon the 17 chapter headings for the International Classification of Diseases:

Table C4   ICD CHAPTER HEADINGS OF BROAD GROUPS
OF CONDITIONS

I : Infective and parasitic diseases.
II : Malignant, benign, lymphatic, haematopoietic and unspecified neoplasms.
III : Endocrine, nutritional and metabolic diseases.
IV : Diseases of blood and blood-forming organs.
V : Mental disorders.
VI : Diseases of nervous system, eye, ear and mastoid process.
VII : Rheumatic fever, hypertensive and heart diseases and diseases of peripheral circulatory system.
VIII : Diseases of respiratory system.
IX : Diseases of digestive system.

X   : Diseases of urinary system, male genital disorders and diseases of breast and female genital system.
XI   : Conditions of pregnancy, childbirth and puerperium.
XII   : Diseases of skin and subcutaneous tissue.
XIII : Diseases of musculoskeletal system and connective tissue.
XIV   : Congenital anomalies.
XV   : Certain causes of perinatal morbidity.
XVI   : Symptoms and ill-defined conditions.
XVII : Other injuries and reactions, fractures, dislocations and sprains.

C7. For each appropriate condition or group of conditions as above, the Regional SMR is multiplied by the age/sex weighted population for that condition and the results aggregated for each Region; the results are then scaled to match the population for England:

Table C5 COMPARISON BY REGION OF POPULATIONS

Crude, and weighted by age/sex non-psychiatric utilisation rates combined with SMRs

Region	Crude population 000s	Weighted population 000s	Ratio of age/sex/SMR weighted population to crude
Northern	3,126.1	3,203	1.02
Yorkshire	3,576.9	3,772	1.05
Trent	4,545.4	4,474	0.98
East Anglian	1,780.4	1,717	0.96
NW Thames	3,475.3	3,246	0.93
NE Thames	3,717.7	3,585	0.96
SE Thames	3,603.2	3,728	1.03
SW Thames	2,880.3	2,922	1.01
Wessex	2,644.9	2,603	0.98
Oxford	2,199.3	1,900	0.86
South Western	3,148.7	3,321	1.05
West Midlands	5,178.1	4,889	0.94
Mersey	2,499.3	2,586	1.03
North Western	4,078.1	4,506	1.10
England	46,453.7	46,452	1.00

Sources: Population – 1975 mid-year estimates; weighting factors from Table C1 and SMRs for 1971.

The algebraic formula for this purpose can be stated as:

Table C6

ALGEBRAIC EXPRESSION FOR PRODUCING POPULATIONS WEIGHTED BY AGE, SEX AND CONDITION SPECIFIC SMRs

$$
\left[\frac{\displaystyle\sum_{i}\sum_{j}\sum_{k} RP_{jk} \cdot \frac{NB_{ijk}}{NP_{jk}} \cdot SMR_{ik}}{\displaystyle\sum_{r}\sum_{i}\sum_{j}\sum_{k} RP_{jk} \cdot \frac{NB_{ijk}}{NP_{jk}} \cdot SMR_{ik}} \right] \left[\sum_{r}\sum_{j}\sum_{k} RP_{rjk} \right]
$$

Where:

NP = national population in year of data on national daily occupied beds
RP = regional population — most recent mid-year estimates
NB = national average number of daily occupied beds
i = condition
j = age group
k = sex
r = region

The first bracket relates to the multiplication of the factors to produce expected bed-days for each Region as a fraction of the total, and the second bracket is the national population which is used to convert the fraction to a weighted population. A comparison of ratios for each Region based on age/sex weights alone and on the combined weighting is as follows:

Table C7 COMPARISON OF RATIOS OF CRUDE POPULATION AND WEIGHTED POPULATION
based on age/sex utilisation rates with and without SMRs

Region	Age/sex utilisation	Age/sex utilisation with SMRs
Northern	0.97	1.02
Yorkshire	1.00	1.05
Trent	0.97	0.98
East Anglian	1.03	0.96
NW Thames	0.97	0.93
NE Thames	1.00	0.96
SE Thames	1.09	1.03
SW Thames	1.06	1.01
Wessex	1.04	0.98
Oxford	0.93	0.86
South Western	1.09	1.05
West Midlands	0.93	0.94
Mersey	0.96	1.03
North Western	1.00	1.10

Sources: Ratios contained in Tables C2 and C5 above.

C8. The conditions for which SMRs are inappropriate are mental disorders (ICD Chapter V), conditions of pregnancy, childbirth and puerperium, (ICD Chapter XI) and diseases of skin and subcutaneous tissue (ICD Chapter XII). For skin conditions (ICD Chapter XII) the value of the SMR for all age/sex groups is set to 100 which means that no additional weight is added to reflect the SMR for this condition, the weighting being determined solely by age and sex. No account is taken of mental illness or handicap in this part of the process – the need for psychiatric services is described later in this Annex. For conditions of pregnancy (ICD Chapter XI) fertility ratios standardised for age are to be applied in a similar way to that in which SMRs are applied for other conditions. These ratios are derived by taking actual births (live and still) as a percentage of 'expected' births, the 'expected' values being calculated by applying the England age-specific (15-24, 25-34, 35-44) fertility rates to the estimated female population in these age bands in each Region. The fertility ratios standardised in this way for each Region to be applied to the female population are set out below but no account has been taken of them in these illustrations:

Table C8   FERTILITY RATIOS FOR EACH REGION STANDARDISED FOR AGE

Region	
Northern	100
Yorkshire	104
Trent	101
East Anglian	105
NW Thames	91
NE Thames	100
SE Thames	97
SW Thames	91
Wessex	102
Oxford	101
South Western	100
West Midlands	103
Mersey	101
North Western	106

Sources: Population – 1974 mid-year estimates; births for 1974.

C9. The figures used in these illustrations have been based on one year's mortality data. The Working Party recommend however that data for as many years as possible be taken subject to a maximum of 10 years (reorganisation of boundaries is the problem in the short term).

C10. *Cost-weighting.* The Working Party recommend that a cost weighting should be applied to the population weighted by the combined factors of age/sex and SMR/SFR. It has not, however, been possible to incorporate such a factor into these illustrative figures. The study referred to in the Report is designed to provide from HIPE data national utilisation rates by age and sex for each group of conditions, as above, but related to hospital type (eg acute, partly acute, orthopaedic, etc). The national costs appropriate to each hospital type published by DHSS would be applied to the data before the multiplication by SMRs. Thus weighted populations would be derived which include a broad measure of known cost differences.

MOVEMENT OF PATIENTS ACROSS ADMINISTRATIVE BOUNDARIES

C11. The weighted populations calculated as above relate to the people living within the administrative boundaries of each Region. Adjustments to the populations either in population terms or through expenditure figures

Table C9   HOSPITAL IN-PATIENT FLOWS ACRO‹
FROM HOSPITAL ACT

Region of Residence (Exporting Authorities)	Northern	Yorkshire	Trent	E Anglian	NW Thames	Regi (Impor NE Thame:
Northern	—	1,795	216	82	207	8⁷
Yorkshire	1,824	—	2,889	161	320	10:
Trent	156	4,500	—	3,089	699	36(
E Anglian	39	64	172	—	1,286	1,28(
NW Thames	87	114	131	1,494	—	10,50‹
NE Thames	67	102	156	1,992	12,371	—
SE Thames	69	86	91	179	6,416	2,59(
SW Thames	51	63	82	150	17,439	2,25‹
Wessex	51	85	80	77	949	33ɛ
Oxford	32	84	165	776	5,526	58ɪ
S Western	50	81	99	92	627	23⁷
W Midlands	110	179	1,578	213	621	21‹
Mersey	114	150	125	42	206	5ɕ
N Western	491	2,222	421	104	224	10⁷
TOTAL CLASSIFIED IMPORTS	3,141	9,525	6,205	8,451	46,891	18,72(
OTHER AND NOT STATED IMPORTS	1,192	744	284	311	3,249	4,324
TOTAL IMPORTS	4,333	10,269	6,489	8,762	50,140	23,044
TOTAL DISCHARGES AND DEATHS from SH3 (excluding maternity and psychiatry)	293,664	338,135	335,546	147,239	341,390	376,914
TOTAL IMPORTS AS A PERCENTAGE OF TOTAL DISCHARGES AND DEATHS	1.5	3.0	1.9	6.0	14.7	6.1
NET FLOW Ratio of Exports to Imports:	1.6:1	0.8:1	3.9:1	0.5:1	0.7:1	0.9:1

NOTES: All figures exclude maternity and psychiatric patients.
*Figures for patients resident in West Midlands but treated in Thames Regions are e
†Figure includes 7,956 from Wales.

eatment thorities) SE Thames	SW Thames	Wessex	Oxford	S Western	W Midlands	Mersey	N Western	Total Exports
298	57	121	112	139	112	210	3,448	6,884
180	104	153	173	234	137	180	1,777	8,235
681	145	239	1,203	383	8,095	181	5,269	25,000
871	174	119	247	126	61	23	52	4,520
7,394	8,495	537	3,530	585	*313	62	121	33,367
4,446	1,144	423	342	316	*46	49	91	21,545
—	12,522	558	347	46	*41	46	88	23,079
15,418	—	1,725	1,727	428	*155	35	87	39,614
431	2,298	—	2,796	3,178	154	63	112	10,612
720	908	1,740	—	381	693	52	94	11,752
434	270	7,413	1,089	—	740	92	112	11,336
169	165	446	742	1,489	—	642	549	7,117
23	68	144	101	279	2,004	—	12,558	15,873
43	89	162	108	380	294	6,411	—	11,056
31,108	26,439	13,780	12,517	7,964	12,845	8,046	24,358	
—	488	1,420	7,166	1,732	240	11,121†	1,534	
31,108	26,927	15,200	19,683	9,696	13,085	19,167	25,892	
350,623	247,420	228,019	197,006	260,427	422,768	232,247	400,839	
8.9	10.9	6.7	10.0	3.7	3.1	8.3	6.5	
0.7:1	1.5:1	0.7:1	0.5:1	1.2:1	0.5:1	0.8:1	0.4:1	

d from one total for all Thames Regions.

are needed to reflect agency arrangements, extra-territorial management arrangements and the referrals of patients to hospitals managed by other Regions. The magnitude of flows resulting from such referrals can be judged from Table C9 which shows the movement of patients between Regions in 1974. All patients referred to the Postgraduate Boards of Governors in London are treated as exports from their Region of residence but are not reflected in the table.

C12.   To compensate and debit Regions for such flows, two factors must be taken into account: the numbers of patients and the cost of providing treatment. Each Region's weighted population is reduced or increased depending upon whether the Region is a net importer or exporter of patients by a notional population adjustment as follows:

C12.1   HAA data are obtained every year from each Region on the numbers of episodes of in-patient treatment by each SH3 specialty incurred by people originating from each of the other 13 Regions and from outside England. Similar data are also obtained from each of the Postgraduate Boards of Governors.

C12.2   The specialty data are aggregated into broad groups of specialties of comparable cost.

C12.3   The net patient flows are derived for each of these groups.

C12.4   The net cost of patient flows for each Region is determined by applying the national average cost per case for each group to the appropriate net flow figures.

C12.5   The resultant adjustments in expenditure terms are converted into population equivalents by reference to the national average cost per head of population on non-psychiatric hospital in-patient services and applied to the appropriate weighted population for each Region.

C13.   The national costs to be attached have been calculated by regression analysis. Several forms of model and several combinations of specialties have been tested starting from the premises that:

C13.1   Length of stay was the major determinant of costs; and

C13.2   The cost per case consisted of two components – a fixed element and a 'per day' element both of which could be varied or fixed for each specialty.

The groupings of specialties and the costs to be attached are shown in Table C10. They were based on a model which assumed that the fixed element varied according to specialty groupings while the 'per day' element remained the same for all specialties.

Table C10 PATIENT FLOWS: SPECIALTY GROUPINGS AND COSTS DERIVED FROM REGRESSION ANALYSIS

The estimated average cost per case for selected groupings of specialties

Cost Group	Estimated Cost Per Case	Standard Error
	£	
1	105	2.7
2	245	15.2
3	369	56.9
4	116	17.3
5	391	19.8
6	91	4.6
7	57	13.9
8	38	29.0
9	156	25.6
10	148	9.5
11	79	4.6
12	114	14.5

Specialties considered	Cost Group	Specialties considered	Cost Group
Cardiology	3	Ophthalmology	6
Convalescent	12	Orthodontics	8
Dental Surgery	8	Orthopaedic Surgery	10
Dermatology	2	Paediatrics	4
Diseases of the Chest	2	Physical Medicine/Rehabilitation	2
ENT	7	Plastic Surgery	9
General Medicine	1	Preconvalescent	12
General Surgery	6	Radiotherapy	9
Geriatric	5	Rheumatology	2
GP Dental	8	Special Baby Care Units	4
GP Maternity	11	Staff Wards	1
GP Others	1	Thoracic Surgery	9
Gynaecology	11	Traumatic and Orthopaedic	
Infectious Diseases	1	Surgery	10
Nephrology	3	Urology	6
Neurology	3	VD	1
Neurosurgery	9	Younger Disabled	5
Obstetrics	11		

Sources: Expenditure from 1971/72 Costing Returns for provincial non-teaching hospitals in types 1 (Acute), 2 (Mainly Acute), and 3 (Partly Acute); Statistics from DHSS Hospital Returns (Form SH3).

C14. The following table reveals the marked difference in the use made of out-patient facilities by men and women of different ages:

Table C11   NATIONAL HOSPITAL DAY- AND OUT-PATIENT ATTENDANCE RATES

by age group and sex in terms of attendances per 1,000 population

Age groups	Males	Females
0– 4	529	560
5–14	619	456
15–44	1,079	1,197
45–64	1,097	1,117
65–74	1,338	1,291
75+	1,101	1,494

Sources: Out-patient attendances derived from the General Household Survey 1971/72 scaled to the national totals by reference to the DHSS Hospital Returns (Form SH3); Population – 1972 mid-year estimates.

The overall SMRs for males and females shown in Table C3 (ie not condition-specific) are recommended for application to this population base in a similar way to that in which the condition-specific SMRs are to be applied to the in-patient services population base. The population breakdown for each Region is multiplied by the national out-patient attendance rates per 1,000 population and further multiplied by the overall sex specific SMRs. The effects of applying the age/sex utilisation rates above and of applying SMRs to the age/sex weighted populations can be seen in the following table:

Table C12   **COMPARISON BY REGION OF**
POPULATIONS

Crude, and weighted by national age/sex rates per 1,000 day and out-patient attendances with and without SMRs

Region	Crude population 000s	Population weighted by age and sex 000s	Population weighted by age, sex and SMRs 000s	Ratio of age/sex/SMR weighted population to crude
Northern	3,126.1	3,110.1	3,404	1.09
Yorkshire	3,576.9	3,569.6	3,764	1.05
Trent	4,545.4	4,521.6	4,609	1.01
East Anglian	1,780.4	1,784.2	1,613	0.91
NW Thames	3,475.3	3,499.6	3,303	0.95
NE Thames	3,717.7	3,736.9	3,602	0.97
SE Thames	3,603.2	3,645.5	3,459	0.96
SW Thames	2,880.3	2,920.9	2,786	0.97
Wessex	2,644.9	2,646.1	2,391	0.90
Oxford	2,199.3	2,169.5	1,950	0.89
South Western	3,148.7	3,186.6	3,040	0.97
West Midlands	5,178.1	5,119.8	5,244	1.01
Mersey	2,499.3	2,471.0	2,767	1.11
North Western	4,078.1	4,072.2	4,519	1.11
England	46,453.7	46,453.6	46,451	1.00

Sources: Population – 1975 mid-year estimates; age/sex weightings from Table C11 and SMRs from Table C3.

C15. *Movement of patients across administrative boundaries.* Only the adjustments to reflect agency arrangements are made in respect of out-patient services.

MEASURING NEED FOR COMMUNITY SERVICES

C16. The following table highlights the differences in usage of community health services made by people of different ages (no split between the sexes is possible):

Table C13   NATIONAL UTILISATION RATES FOR COMMUNITY HEALTH SERVICES

by age group in terms of expenditure per 1,000 population

Age groups	£
0– 4	15.32
5–14	7.36
15–64	0.67
65 and over	7.15

Sources: Population – 1971 mid-year estimates; expenditure from local health authorities' returns for 1971/72.

As for out-patient services, the Working Party recommend that populations and age/sex weights should be adjusted to take into account overall SMRs for each Region; the following table shows populations weighted in this way:

Table C14 COMPARISON BY REGION OF POPULATIONS

Crude, and weighted by national community health services expenditure rates with and without SMRs

Region	Crude population 000s	Population weighted by age and sex 000s	Population weighted by age, sex and SMRs 000s	Ratio of age/sex/SMR weighted population to crude
Northern	3,126.1	3,111.0	3,404	1.09
Yorkshire	3,576.9	3,629.9	3,825	1.07
Trent	4,545.4	4,546.2	4,631	1.02
East Anglian	1,780.4	1,812.6	1,638	0.92
NW Thames	3,475.3	3,270.8	3,086	0.89
NE Thames	3,717.7	3,651.5	3,518	0.95
SE Thames	3,603.2	3,646.6	3,459	0.96
SW Thames	2,880.3	2,823.7	2,692	0.93
Wessex	2,644.9	2,715.8	2,453	0.93
Oxford	2,199.3	2,203.9	1,980	0.90
South Western	3,148.7	3,192.5	3,044	0.97
West Midlands	5,178.1	5,165.9	5,289	1.02
Mersey	2,499.3	2,537.0	2,839	1.14
North Western	4,078.1	4,146.4	4,599	1.13
England	46,453.7	46,453.8	46,457	1.00

Sources: Population – 1975 mid-year estimates; age/sex weightings from Table C13 and SMRs from Table C3.

C17. *Movement of patients across administrative boundaries.* Only the adjustments to reflect agency arrangements are made in respect of community health services.

MEASURING NEED FOR AMBULANCE SERVICES

C18. Crude populations are recommended as the basic determinant of need for ambulance services but some measure of morbidity is thought necessary since demands must be affected by morbidity levels. SMRs should, therefore, be used in the same way as for other community services. The effect on each Region's crude population is as follows:

Table C15 COMPARISON BY REGION OF POPULATIONS
Crude and weighted by SMRs

Region	Crude population 000s	Population weighted by SMRs 000s	Ratio of SMR weighted population to crude
Northern	3,126.1	3,376	1.08
Yorkshire	3,576.9	3,741	1.05
Trent	4,545.4	4,619	1.02
East Anglian	1,780.4	1,635	0.92
NW Thames	3,475.3	3,309	0.95
NE Thames	3,717.7	3,603	0.97
SE Thames	3,603.2	3,446	0.96
SW Thames	2,880.3	2,767	0.96
Wessex	2,644.9	2,428	0.92
Oxford	2,199.3	2,010	0.91
South Western	3,148.7	3,025	0.96
West Midlands	5.178.1	5,284	1.02
Mersey	2,499.3	2,753	1.10
North Western	4,078.1	4,457	1.09
England	46,453.7	46,453	1.00

Sources: Population – 1975 mid-year estimates; SMRs from Table C3.

MEASURING NEED FOR MENTAL ILLNESS SERVICES

C19. As for non-psychiatric in-patients there are clear differences in usage of mental illness beds between people of different ages and of each sex:

Table C16 NATIONAL HOSPITAL MENTAL ILLNESS UTILISATION RATES

by age group for each sex in terms of bed-days per 1,000 population

Age groups	Males	Females
0–14	28	17
15–19	122	140
20–24	267	232
25–34	373	286
35–44	558	429
45–64	1,167	903
65–74	1,604	1,976
75+	2,320	3,897

Sources: Population – 1974 mid-year estimates; bed-days from 1974 MHE data.

There are however also marked differences in utilisation between the married and non-married as the following table shows. The Working Party accordingly recommended that marital status be introduced as an added dimension to the population base for mental illness services:

Table C17 NATIONAL HOSPITAL PSYCHIATRIC (MENTAL ILLNESS) IN-PATIENT SERVICES

Proportion of Mental Illness Residents by age group and marital status for each sex

Age groups	Males		Females	
	Married	Non-Married	Married	Non-Married
	%	%	%	%
15–19	0.98	99.02	4.18	95.82
20–24	4.88	95.12	21.98	78.02
25–34	13.52	86.48	37.91	62.09
35–44	16.02	83.98	37.77	62.23
45–54	15.15	84.85	29.98	70.02
55–64	21.40	78.60	25.30	74.70
65–74	26.69	73.31	21.30	78.70
75 and over	29.09	70.91	12.47	87.53

Source: Census of Patients in Mental Illness Hospitals and Units in England and Wales, 31 December 1971.

The national utilisation rates will be produced in such a way as to reflect these differences and be applied to the appropriate characteristics of each Region's population (ie age, sex and marital status) by simple multiplication and scaling as for other population bases. For the purposes of these illustrations however, only the age/sex differences have been reflected into the following weighted populations:

Table C18 **COMPARISON BY REGION OF POPULATIONS**

Crude, and weighted by national age/sex mental illness in-patient utilisation rates

Region	Crude population 000s	Population weighted by age and sex 000s	Ratio of age/sex weighted population to crude
Northern	3,126.1	3,071.8	0.98
Yorkshire	3,576.9	3,590.7	1.00
Trent	4,545.4	4,461.1	0.98
East Anglian	1,780.4	1,766.2	0.99
NW Thames	3,475.3	3,417.1	0.98
NE Thames	3,717.7	3,763.6	1.01
SE Thames	3,603.2	3,867.5	1.07
SW Thames	2,880.3	3,070.2	1.07
Wessex	2,644.9	2,636.3	1.00
Oxford	2,199.3	1,991.4	0.91
South Western	3,148.7	3,367.3	1.07
West Midlands	5,178.1	4,904.5	0.95
Mersey	2,499.3	2,404.5	0.96
North Western	4,078.1	4,141.5	1.02
England	4,6453.7	46,453.7	1.00

Sources: Population – 1975 mid-year estimates; age/sex weighting from Table C16.

MEASURING NEED FOR MENTAL HANDICAP SERVICES

C20. As for other services, there is a clear difference in utilisation rates between the age/sex groups as the following table demonstrates:

Table C19   NATIONAL HOSPITAL PSYCHIATRIC (MENTAL HANDICAP) IN-PATIENT UTILISATION RATES
by age group for each sex in terms of bed-days per 1,000 population

Age groups	Males	Females
0– 4	30	25
5–14	243	166
15–19	576	359
20–24	583	403
25–34	619	437
35–44	576	451
45–64	519	475
65–74	441	373
75 and over	241	217

Sources: Population – 1974 mid-year estimates; bed-days from 1974 MHE data.

And these national rates are applied to the crude population of each Region in the same way as for other population bases – no other factors can be added at present:

Table C20   COMPARISON BY REGION OF POPULATIONS
Crude, and weighted by national age/sex mental handicap in-patient utilisation rates

Region	Crude population 000s	Population weighted by age and sex 000s	Ratio of age/sex weighted population to crude
Northern	3,126.1	3,140.2	1.00
Yorkshire	3,576.9	3,570.5	1.00
Trent	4,545.4	4,550.4	1.00
East Anglian	1,780.4	1,741.6	0.98
NW Thames	3,475.3	3,521.2	1.01
NE Thames	3,717.7	3,751.2	1.01
SE Thames	3,603.2	3,622.3	1.01
SW Thames	2,880.3	2,922.1	1.01
Wessex	2,644.9	2,586.5	0.98
Oxford	2,199.3	2,147.4	0.98
South Western	3,148.7	3,142.7	1.00
West Midlands	5,178.1	5,179.0	1.00
Mersey	2,499.3	2,485.8	0.99
North Western	4,078.1	4,092.8	1.00
England	46,453.7	46,453.7	1.00

Sources: Population – 1975 mid-year estimates; age/sex weightings from Table C19.

114

MOVEMENT OF PSYCHIATRIC PATIENTS ACROSS ADMINISTRATIVE BOUNDARIES (BOTH MENTAL ILLNESS AND MENTAL HANDICAP)

C21. The recommendations in the Report to reflect agency arrangements, patient flows etc are effected in a similar way to that described for acute services except that no costs can be attached. The assumption therefore is that the cost of treating each psychiatric patient who crosses an administrative boundary is the same in all cases. Total numbers of net exports or imports are converted into notional population adjustments by reference to the total national number of psychiatric in-patient cases per head of population.

C.22 The adjustment for long-stay patients whose length of stay exceeded one year when the last censuses of mental illness and mental handicap took place is effected by means of a comparison between actual numbers in each Region and those which would be expected based on age/sex national utilisation rates. This process can be described as follows:

C22.1 The years of the last censuses (1971 for mental illness, 1970 for mental handicap) are chosen as the base years. *Actual numbers* are known from these data for each Region, and *expected numbers* are calculated by applying to the age/sex structure of each Region's population the national average numbers in each age/sex group of long-stay mental illness and mental handicap patients per head of population in the base years.

C22.2 The next stage, which needs to be recalculated every year, takes account of the rates of decline for these groups of patients since the base years: *actual numbers* for each Region are updated from the latest available data and *expected numbers* are adjusted by reference to the national reduction in the numbers of such patients since the base years as revealed in these latest available data. The *actual* and *expected* figures are further projected to the years of allocation by reference to the national rates of decline of these patients (9% for mental illness and 7% for mental handicap).

C22.3 Notional Regional deficits or surpluses of these patients are determined by subtracting the expected from the estimated actual numbers of patients.

C22.4 The net cost of treatment of the deficits or surpluses of each Region is derived by multiplying by the appropriate national average

Table C21   1975 POPULATION WEIGHTED FOR REVENUE PURPOSES

1975 Mid-year Estimates of Population (000s)

Weighted to reflect revenue need for services for

Region	Crude Population	Non-psychiatric In-Patients	All Day and Out-patients	Community Health	Ambulances	Mental Illness In-patients	Mental Handicap In-patients	FPC Administration	Aggregated Weighted Population
1. Northern	3126.1	3203	3404	3404	3376	3071.8	3140.2	3126.1	3233.7
2. Yorkshire	3576.9	3772	3764	3825	3741	3590.7	3570.5	3576.9	3740.2
3. Trent	4545.4	4474	4609	4631	4619	4461.1	4550.4	4545.4	4514.4
4. East Anglian	1780.4	1717	1613	1638	1635	1766.2	1741.6	1780.4	1700.9
5. NW Thames	3475.3	3246	3303	3086	3309	3417.1	3521.2	3475.3	3279.7
6. NE Thames	3717.7	3585	3602	3518	3603	3763.6	3751.2	3717.7	3614.0
7. SE Thames	3603.2	3728	3459	3459	3446	3867.5	3622.3	3603.2	3668.8
8. SW Thames	2880.3	2922	2786	2692	2767	3070.2	2922.1	2880.3	2896.1
9. Wessex	2644.9	2603	2391	2453	2428	2636.3	2586.5	2644.9	2558.8
10. Oxford	2199.3	1900	1950	1980	2010	1991.4	2147.4	2199.3	1944.3
11. South Western	3148.7	3321	3040	3044	3025	3367.3	3142.7	3148.7	3243.2
12. West Midlands	5178.1	4889	5244	5289	5284	4904.5	5179.0	5178.1	5005.5
13. Mersey	2499.3	2586	2767	2839	2753	2404.5	2485.8	2499.3	2610.1
14. North Western	4078.1	4506	4519	4599	4457	4141.5	4092.8	4078.1	4444.0
England	46453.7	46452	46451	46457	46453	46453.7	46453.7	46453.7	46453.7

Estimated National Proportions of Revenue Expenditure on each Service:

		55.9%	13.4%	8.8%	3.5%	12.2%	5.7%	0.5%	100%

cost per year of long-stay mental handicap and mental illness patients and summing the two resulting component costs; finally these costs are converted to notional corrections to the population of each Region by dividing by the national expenditure per head of population on long stay psychiatric patients.

For the purposes of the illustrations in the Report, a limited form of this adjustment has been made, which takes no account of the rate of decline for each of these groups of patients.

ESTABLISHING THE TARGETS FOR RHAs

C.23   Table C21 shows how the recommendation for combining the seven separate weighted populations is put into effect for each RHA. Before the total revenue for services can be apportioned between RHAs in relation to the 14 aggregated weighted populations, adjustments must be made to reflect:

   i   agency arrangements
   ii patient flows
   iii the numbers of long-stay psychiatric patients
   iv London Weighting.

These adjustments have been calculated for each weighted population and Table C22 demonstrates the distribution of revenue funds between Regions on the basis of *adjusted* weighted populations.

Table C22 DISTRIBUTION OF NATIONAL REVENUE FUNDS FOR SERVICES IN PROPORTION TO AGGREGATED WEIGHTED POPULATION

Region	Adjusted Weighted Population 000s	Revenue Funds for Services £000s
Northern	3,183.4	160,814
Yorkshire	3,679.7	186,485
Trent	4,320.1	212,772
East Anglian	1,677.5	88,664
NW Thames	3,355.4	211,315
NE Thames	3,719.1	235,112
SE Thames	3,843.3	225,163
SW Thames	3,132.2	178,920
Wessex	2,581,2	131,240
Oxford	1,925.8	105,905
South Western	3,032.2	159,201
West Midlands	4,941.0	252,738
Mersey	2,606.1	137,848
North Western	4,456.9	219,086
England	46,453.9	2,505,263

Sources: Weighted populations from Table C21 adjusted for factors at C23 i – iv; total revenue funds for services for 1977/78 at March 1975 prices assuming 1½% growth.

DISTRIBUTION OF CAPITAL FUNDS TO REGIONAL HEALTH AUTHORITIES

VALUING THE STOCK AND WEIGHTING THE POPULATION

D1. This annex gives more details about the Working Party's recommendations for valuing the existing capital stock in the NHS both Regionally and nationally and weighting the population to assess each RHA's relative need for capital.

VALUING THE STOCK

D2. The valuation method adopted combines an assessment of stock values as at 1961 with aggregate adjusted capital expenditure since that date in order to reflect renewal and upgrading as well as new building. Although the term capital stock is deemed to cover all NHS buildings and all equipment charged to capital, numbers of beds have been used as a proxy for hospital capital stock up to 1961. The stock is first valued according to its 1975 replacement cost. This cost is an 'all-in' cost which reflects all supporting services (including out-patient departments and their back-up facilities) in terms of the costs of works, fees, furniture, equipment and residences but not of land. This value of stock is then 'written down' to reflect its age and condition. The process is as follows:

D2.1 Each RHB's average available stock of beds, plus the appropriate undergraduate hospital beds situated in each RHB, as at 31 December 1961, is valued at 1975 replacement cost.

D2.2 This value of stock for each RHB is then 'written down' by factors appropriate to each RHB.

D2.3 To these values of beds as at 1961 is added RHB (and RHA) and relevant BG (ie Undergraduate Teaching Hospitals) capital expenditure from 1962/63 to 1975/76 inclusive and 1976/77 allocations.

D2.4 Certain adjustments are made to the above estimates of RHB and BG stocks, to allow for changes since 1961 and the reorganization of 1974.

D3. *Calculation of 'Bed Replacement Costs'*. The broad distinction in terms of capital costs of providing beds and the necessary back-up facilities (as defined in paragraph D2 above) is between the short-stay specialties (acute) and the long-stay specialties (non-acute). Non-acute beds comprise the SH3 specialties of Geriatrics, Chronic Sick, Mental Illness – Children, Subnormality and Severe Subnormality (ie Mental Handicap), Mental Illness and Chronic Sick under Psychiatric Supervision. Acute beds are any beds not counted as above. Acute bed capital costs were derived from information on a theoretical DGH, typical of actual DGH building schemes. DGHs exclude non-acute beds as defined above; they include, however, geriatric acute/assessment beds but these are not the kind of beds denoted by the Geriatric Specialty in 1961. The cost of a bed in DGH was therefore taken as the cost of an acute bed and this has been assessed at £24,000 at 1975 Cost Allowance level, inclusive of on-costs, fees and equipment. For non-acute beds the cost of a bed based on Cost Allowances for a 150-bedded community hospital has been taken: this is £12,000. (1975 Cost Allowances, inclusive of on-costs, fees and equipment.)

D4. *Calculation of Depreciation Factors*. There are two features to the production of such factors:

D4.1 Firstly proportion of floor area in each Region (RHB including relevant Undergraduate Teaching Hospitals) in particular age categories had to be determined from information in the 1972 Hospital Maintenance Survey – the categories being pre-1918, 1919-48, 1949-61. For each (RHB) Region total floor area was estimated by grossing up from the floor area of hospitals responding to the Hospital Maintenance Survey, on the basis of the number of beds in each Region (SH3 1971 information) relative to the number of beds in the responding hospitals. For each individual Region, therefore, the floor area per bed including supporting services was assumed to be the same for responding and non-responding hospitals. Teaching hospital floor area was similarly, but separately, grossed-up and allocated to Regions in proportion to the number of teaching hospital beds in each Region. Age profiles were obtained by allocating the undated floor areas in the same proportions as dated floor areas. (This was done separately for London Teaching, Provincial Teaching and RHB hospitals.) Teaching and non-teaching floor areas in each age category were summed for each Region. Since these data recorded floor areas for the whole of the period 1949-72, floor area for 1949-61 had to be estimated by reference to the capital spent in each Region between 1949-61 as a proportion of that spent between 1949-72; all expenditure figures were revalued to 1975 price levels.

D4.2 Secondly, percentage depreciation factors for each of the three periods were calculated by analysing DGH costs to obtain approximate percentage costs attributable to the various elements of a hospital (walls, floors, etc). These elements were then considered to see how they would depreciate over time and approximate percentage depreciation factors were ascribed. These were then weighted by the cost attributed to each element and an overall weighted depreciation factor calculated: the results were: 1949-61 – 50%; 1919-48 – 65%; pre-1918 – 70%. The effect on these overall results of varying the depreciation factors related to the various elements of hospital construction was tested but found to be insignificant.

D5. These depreciation factors were applied to floor area proportions for each Region and a weighted average depreciation factor produced for each Region. Table D1 provides details of proportions of floor area by RHB in each category and the weighted average depreciation factors in terms of 'Remaining Value', ie as a coefficient of 1975 replacement cost:

Table D1 FLOOR AREA PROPORTIONS IN EACH AGE CATEGORY AND WEIGHTED AVERAGE DEPRECIATION FACTORS FOR 1961 STOCK

Region	Proportions of floor area in			Weighted Average Depreciation Factor
	Pre-1918 %	1919-48 %	1949-61 (est) %	
Newcastle	50.07	35.71	14.22	.3463
Leeds	63.94	28.95	7.11	.3287
Sheffield	58.22	32.20	9.58	.3353
East Anglian	66.19	24.93	8.88	.3303
NW Met	65.47	28.94	5.59	.3257
NE Met	61.05	34.04	4.91	.3269
SE Met	74.21	22.10	3.69	.3185
SW Met	71.85	22.07	6.08	.3232
Oxford	49.20	41.50	9.30	.3394
South Western	57.87	34.41	7.72	.3326
Birmingham	63.30	30.37	6.33	.3279
Manchester	69.80	24.15	6.05	.3242
Liverpool	76.35	18.84	4.81	.3191
Wessex	67.42	29.81	2.77	.3205
England	64.96	28.43	6.61	.3275

Sources: Hospital Maintenance Survey 1972; DHSS Hospital Returns (Form SH3); depreciation factors derived by DHSS.

This factor was used to 'write down' the 1975 cost of the beds of each hospital existing in 1961 – it was thus an average 'write-down' showing the percentage amount by which the average bed including supporting services in each individual Region would have been depreciated if nothing had been done to it between 1961 and 1975. The factors produced showed that, for example, the average hospital in England in 1961 would have been worth in 1975 only 32.75% of its 1975 replacement cost if nothing had been done to improve it or replace its engineering services etc since 1961.

D6. *RHB (and RHA) and BG Capital Expenditure 1962-1976 and 1976-77 allocation.* Capital expenditure* including works, fees, equipment, furniture, capitalised maintenance and from 1974/75 expenditure on purchase of land incurred by Authorities from 1962/63 to 1975/76 inclusive and allocations for 1976/77 (including additional resources from land sales etc) were added to the 1975 cost of beds written down as above in order to reflect renewal, upgrading and new building. The figures were revalued to 1975 price levels and depreciated at a rate of 2.4% per annum – a rate derived directly from the 50% write-down used for the 1949-61 period. Undergraduate Teaching Hospital expenditure was included at 65% except in relation to 1975/76 where details were not available.

D7. *Adjustments to reflect changes since 1961.* The following adjustments were made where appropriate to each Region's total value of stock:

D7.1   Closures. Hospitals closed between 1961 and March 1974 were valued in the same way as above, ie by costing beds and adding post-1961 depreciated capital expenditure. The values of closed hospitals were subtracted from the Regional figures. Closures of hospitals occurring between April 1974 and March 1976, together with agreed future closures were taken account of by costing their 1961 beds at depreciated 1975 replacement costs, but it was not possible to exclude capital expenditure since 1961 on such hospitals.

D7.2   Downgrading. Hospitals which were of Types 1 to 3 in 1961 (Acute, Mainly Acute, Partly Acute) but which had been reclassified by 1974 were deemed to have been downgraded. Their values were decreased by the amount of the decreased values of their acute beds.

---

*For a full definition of capital expenditure, see DS 266/72 as adjusted by DS 57/74 (to include land acquisition from 1 April 1974) and further amended by the 1976/77 allocation letter dated 18 February 1976 by which the thresholds were revised.

D7.3 'Cottage Hospitals'. Cottage hospitals were defined as being hospitals with fewer than 100 beds classified as acute but mostly controlled by GPs, and having no pathology facilities. Acute beds in such hospitals were counted and valued at the lower (non-acute) replacement cost.

D7.4 Regional Transfers. Hospitals which were transferred from the management of one Region to another on reorganisation were valued by the 'beds plus expenditure' method (but allowing for possible 'cottage' or 'downgrading' elements) and their values transferred between the Regions. In all transfers the depreciation factors used were those appropriate to the Region in which the hospital was situated before reorganisation.

D7.5 Ex-Local Authority Health Premises. It was originally hoped that rateable values could be used in the valuation of ex-Local Authority premises. However, consistent lists of, and rateable values for, these premises have not been available from all RHAs. In addition it was doubtful whether a formula could have been devised that could be applied to rateable value to obtain a capital value for such diverse premises as health centres and ambulance stations. A much restricted proxy had to be used, namely the number of health centres in each Region at end-March 1974, costed at 1975 replacement cost (at a figure per GP accommodated of £24,800 which also took account of other primary care services). Data deficiencies prevented the valuation of other ex-Local Authority property such as ambulance stations and offices.

D8. The result of all the operations described above is the estimated value of RHA capital stocks, at 1975 price levels, as at end-March 1977 and Table D2 quantifies each of the processes involved. The following additional points should be noted:

D8.1 Joint user premises, non-NHS premises in which contractual arrangements are provided and private practice GP premises were not taken into account.

D8.2 Private beds in NHS hospitals were included in Regional bed stocks.

D8.3 Undergraduate Teaching Hospital beds were valued at the same rate as non-teaching beds.

Table D2

VALUATION OF EXISTING CAPITAL STOCK BY REGION

£000s at 1975 Prices

Region	Corresponding RHB Value (March 1974) including Undergraduate Teaching Hospitals	Value of Closures Since 1961 (−)	Value of Transfers Out (−)	Value of Transfers In (+)	Adjustment for Downgraded and Cottage Hospital Acute Beds (−)	Trust Funds Expenditure 1966/7 – 1973/4 (+)	Value of Health Centres (at end-March 1974) (+)	RHA Capital Expenditure 1974/5 – 76/7 (+)	RHA Capital Stock (March 1977)
	(1)	(2)	(3)	(4)	(5)	(6)	(7)	(8)	(9)
Northern	301,252	10,699	3,507	9,682	5,394	2,113	6,291	61,854	361,592
Yorkshire	335,302	20,496	441	20,293	5,632	2,372	4,953	71,605	407,956
Trent	410,685	17,437	16,786	1,414	5,923	2,323	7,764	108,544	490,584
East Anglian	181,797	3,884	1,248	—	2,778	771	1,350	42,501	218,509
NW Thames	457,902	7,069	115,103	47,338	5,436	1,491	2,737	65,741	447,601
NE Thames	335,310	6,244	1,944	81,770	4,516	3,309	3,121	70,230	481,036
SE Thames	337,732	10,967	10,118	42,493	3,746	10,961	1,436	72,276	440,067
SW Thames	381,045	839	89,605	18,690	5,978	875	3,418	69,110	376,716
Wessex	186,322	3,915	—	50,527	6,625	834	3,863	54,830	285,836
Oxford	206,194	3,833	21,594	25,783	3,137	3,474	2,984	56,423	266,294
South Western	334,487	6,027	31,607	2,674	9,292	1,443	7,033	62,289	361,000
West Midlands	462,558	4,445	—	—	6,071	2,050	6,761	94,396	555,249
Mersey	262,663	5,969	5,119	40,690	6,513	522	2,910	61,307	350,491
North Western	410,182	2,704	51,345	5,119	5,533	2,396	6,006	81,553	445,674
England (excl. Postgraduate BGs)	4,603,431	104,528	348,417	346,473	76,574	34,934	60,627	972,659	5,488,605

NOTE: Cols (3) and (4): discrepancy between totals (£1,944,000) is accounted for by transfers from RHAs into the Postgraduate Boards of Governors.

D8.4   Hospitals not under the control of RHAs – eg independent and charitable institutions, Service hospitals and Postgraduate (preserved) Boards of Governors (BGs) – were not counted in any Region's stock. In many of these cases, use of services by NHS patients is paid for by the RHA, or subject to 'knock for knock' arrangements, or is not significantly different between Regions. This is not, however, the case with the Postgraduate BGs, which draw a very substantial proportion of their patients from four Regions. An adjustment is made to revenue allocations to take account of care received in BGs, and there could well be a case for charging their capitalised maintenance costs also to those Regions which are major users of their facilities, in proportion to the service received. The future of the BGs is however at present under consideration and, in view of possible changes in the management of some or all BGs, consideration of this issue should be deferred until the picture is clearer.

D8.5   Trust Funds expenditure before 1974 has been included.

WEIGHTING THE POPULATION

D9.   This part of the annex describes how the Working Party's proposals for weighting the population for capital distribution purposes can be implemented: the methodology follows closely that recommended for revenue and is, therefore, described in less detail. There are, however, some important changes referred to in the Report; these are:

D9.1   *Population base.* A population projection five years ahead of the year for which allocations are to be made is recommended for the reasons set out in the Report.

D9.2   *Non-psychiatric in-patient services.* The same variation in age/sex utilisation rates and in SMRs and SFRs which led the Working Party to the conclusions in Chapter II (Tables C1-C7 of Annex C) also apply to capital. The methodology and data are precisely the same as for revenue.

D9.3   *Day- and out-patient services.* As for revenue the population should be weighted by age/sex utilisation in terms of out-patient attendances per 1,000 population (as derived from the General Household Survey 1971/72/73 and scaled to the national total by reference to the DHSS Hospital Return (Form SH3)) and adjusted by overall sex-specific Regional SMRs.

D9.4 *Community services*. As the report states the age weights used for revenue are not considered appropriate for capital and a better measure is thought to be GP consultation rates (excluding telephone conversations and visits to patients' homes) by age and sex based on data from the General Household Survey aggregated for three years, 1971/72/73. The population should be modified further by the overall Regional SMRs. Table D3 shows a comparison between crude population and population weighted by age and sex for capital for community services:

Table D3   COMPARISON BY REGION OF POPULATIONS

Crude, and weighted by reference to national GP consultation rates by age and sex

Region	Crude population 000s	Weighted population 000s	Ratio of weighted to crude population
Northern	3,172.7	3,049.0	0.961
Yorkshire	3,576.1	3,583.8	1.002
Trent	4,661.4	4,661.9	1.000
East Anglian	1,897.5	1,901.3	1.002
NW Thames	3,584.0	3,613.2	1.008
NE Thames	3,873.6	3,900.7	1.007
SE Thames	3,748.4	3,782.6	1.009
SW Thames	2,917.7	2,949.8	1.011
Wessex	2,815.9	2,819.2	1.001
Oxford	2,403.4	2,384.7	0.992
South Western	3,250.0	3,279.8	1.009
West Midlands	5,341.8	5,320.9	0.996
Mersey	2,542.8	2,525.5	0.993
North Western	4,145.6	4,158.5	1.003
England	47,930.9	47,930.9	1.000

Sources: Population-1981 projection (1971-based); GP consultation rates from General Household Survey 1971.

D9.5 *Psychiatric services*. For mental illness, age, sex and marital status should be used and for mental handicap, age and sex alone. No adjustment is made for the old long-stay psychiatric patients.

D9.6 *Ambulance and FPC administration*. A weighted population for ambulance services is produced in exactly the same way as for revenue but no population base is produced for FPC administration.

D10. *Aggregated weighted populations.* The six separate weighted populations for each Region are combined to form a single weighted population for each. Table D4 shows how this is done based on estimated national proportions of capital spending (ie capital expenditure as defined in paragraph D6) on the services concerned for the next three years. The same factors which could not be included in the revenue illustrations have also not been reflected into the populations weighted for capital purposes.

Table D4 1981 WEIGHTED POPULATION TO BE USED FOR
(a) DETERMINING CAPITAL ALLOCATIONS AND (b) ASSESSING
TARGETS IN TERMS OF STOCK VALUATIONS

		1981 *projected population (1971-based) 000s*					
		Weighted to reflect capital need for services for					
Region	*Crude*	*Non-psychiatric in-patients*	*All day- and out-patients*	*Psychiatric in-patients*	*Community health*	*Ambulances*	*Aggregated Weighted population*
Northern	3,172.7	3,253.7	3,472.1	3,131.7	3,341.9	3,475.5	3,276.0
Yorkshire	3,576.1	3,775.1	3,779.8	3,592.4	3,783.4	3,773.7	3,749.8
Trent	4,661.4	4,563.9	4,697.7	4,535.2	4,726.7	4,754.6	4,593.9
East Anglian	1,897.5	1,831.4	1,714.6	1,913.9	1,720.7	1,716.3	1,817.1
NW Thames	3,584.0	3,379.1	3,440.5	3,588.1	3,443.1	3,385.0	3,422.4
NE Thames	3,873.6	3,738.6	3,747.1	3,843.2	3,762.3	3,737.3	3,756.5
SE Thames	3,748.4	3,881.7	3,588.3	3,867.1	3,633.1	3,559.9	3,815.1
SW Thames	2,917.7	3,091.6	2,953.2	3,183.1	2,939.1	2,787.5	3,068.3
Wessex	2,815.9	2,802.4	2,583.2	2,952.9	2,576.7	2,548.2	2,772.8
Oxford	2,403.4	2,078.0	2,122.3	2,261.9	2,145.8	2,161.7	2,117.6
South Western	3,250.0	3,235.3	2,963.7	3,299.0	2,955.5	3,102.0	3,184.9
West Midlands	5,341.8	5,048.5	5,422.8	5,149.7	5,457.0	5,475.8	5,152.7
Mersey	2,542.8	2,633.2	2,832.8	2,465.2	2,825.5	2,849.4	2,654.5
North Western	4,145.6	4,618.4	4,612.8	4,147.5	4,620.1	4,604.0	4,549.3
England	47,930.9	47,930.9	47,930.9	47,930.9	47,930.9	47,930.9	47,930.9

Estimated National Proportional Capital Spending on each Service:

	62.6%	12.9%	14.5%	7.7%	2.3%	100%

The first two years' figures on proportional spending were based on the forward estimates supplied by each Region and the third year's estimate was derived from the capital projections given in the Consultative Document on Priorities for Health and Personal Social Services in England. The proportions including those from the Consultative Document should be up-dated every year based on the latest three years' estimates. The proportional expenditure on out-patient services was calculated by DHSS.

D11. Weighted populations are used by themselves to distribute part of the total available capital each year and, in combination with the valuation of total capital stock, to determine those Regions who fall short of their targets and require additional funds. Table D5 illustrates the relationship for each Region between the actual capital stock value and that based on a notional distribution of the total capital wealth in the NHS:

Table D5   COMPARISON OF EXISTING CAPITAL STOCK VALUES WITH TARGETS REPRESENTING NOTIONAL DISTRIBUTION OF TOTAL CAPITAL WEALTH

Region	RHA capital stock value (March 1977) £000s	Target based on notional distribution £000s	Shortfall/Excess per head of weighted population £	Amounts required to rectify shortfalls £000s
Northern	361,592	375,137	4.13 (S)	13,545
Yorkshire	407,956	429,393	5.72 (S)	21,437
Trent	490,584	526,051	7.72 (S)	35,467
East Anglian	218,509	208,078	5.74 (E)	—
NW Thames	447,601	391,902	16.28 (E)	—
NE Thames	481,036	430,160	13.54 (E)	—
SE Thames	440,067	436,870	0.84 (E)	—
SW Thames	376,716	351,353	8.27 (E)	—
Wessex	285,836	317,515	11.42 (S)	31,679
Oxford	266,294	242,488	11.24 (E)	—
South Western	361,000	364,705	1.16 (S)	3,705
West Midlands	555,249	590,040	6.75 (S)	34,791
Mersey	350,491	303,969	17.53 (E)	—
North Western	445,674	520,944	16.54 (S)	75,270
Totals	5,488,605	5,488,604	—	215,894

D12. The methods for determining actual allocations are fully described in the Report; the flow chart (Figure D1) shows this process in diagrammatic form, and Table D6 sets out in summary form for each year the proportions of available capital for distribution on a weighted population and on a shortfall element basis:

APPLICATION OF THE CAPITAL DISTRIBUTION FORMULA TO PRODUCE CAPITAL ALLOCATIONS

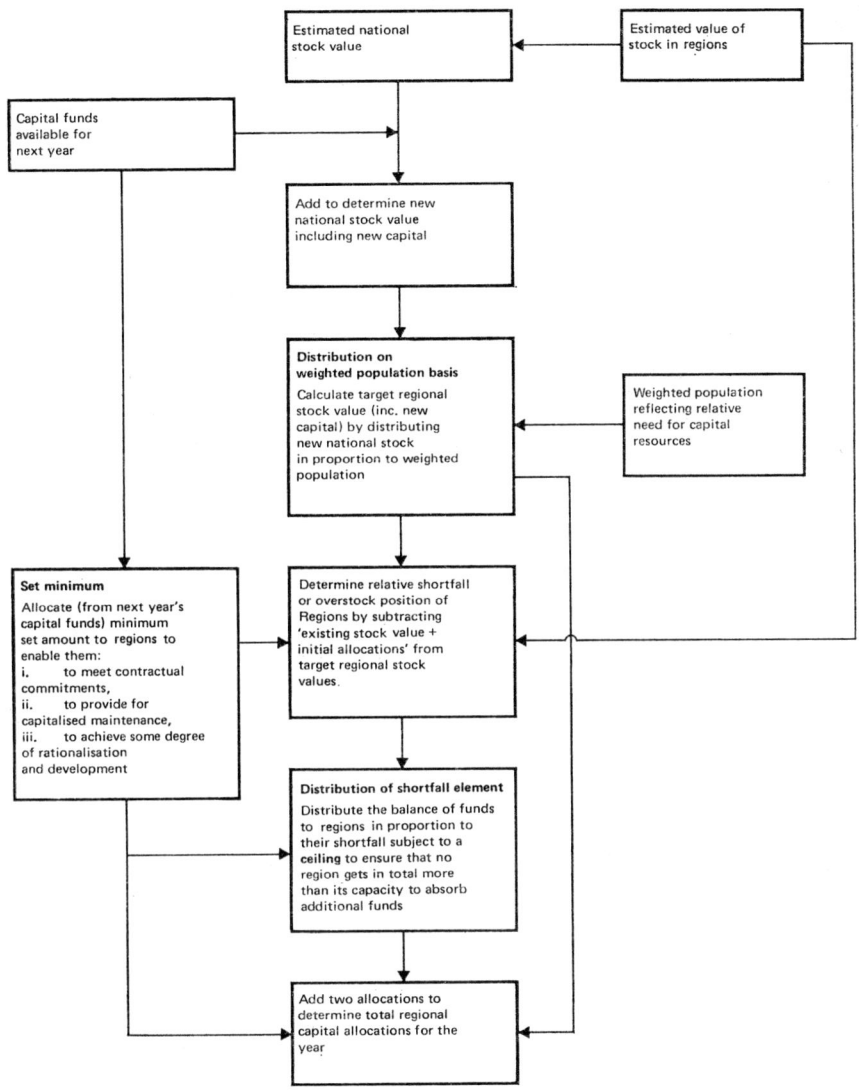

Table D6   **PROPORTIONS OF CAPITAL FUNDS**
AVAILABLE FOR DISTRIBUTION EACH YEAR

Year	The minimum level based on planning assumptions in first two years and weighted population thereafter	The proportion of funds for the shortfall element	The 'ceiling' setting based on percentage of all capital distributed on weighted population
1977/78	90%	10%	110%
1978/79	80%	20%	120%
1979/80	70%	30%	130%
1980/81	70%	30%	140%
1981/82	70%	30%	140%
1982/83	80%	20%	140%
1983/84	80%	20%	140%
1984/85	80%	20%	140%
1985/86	90%	10%	140%
1986/87	90%	10%	140%

D13.   Figures D2 and D3 show over the next 10 years an illustrative pattern of allocations for each RHA (Figure D2) and the position each would have achieved in relation to its target by the year 1987 (Figure D3).

TIME PROFILE OF ILLUSTRATIVE CAPITAL ALLOCATIONS
OVER A TEN YEAR PERIOD

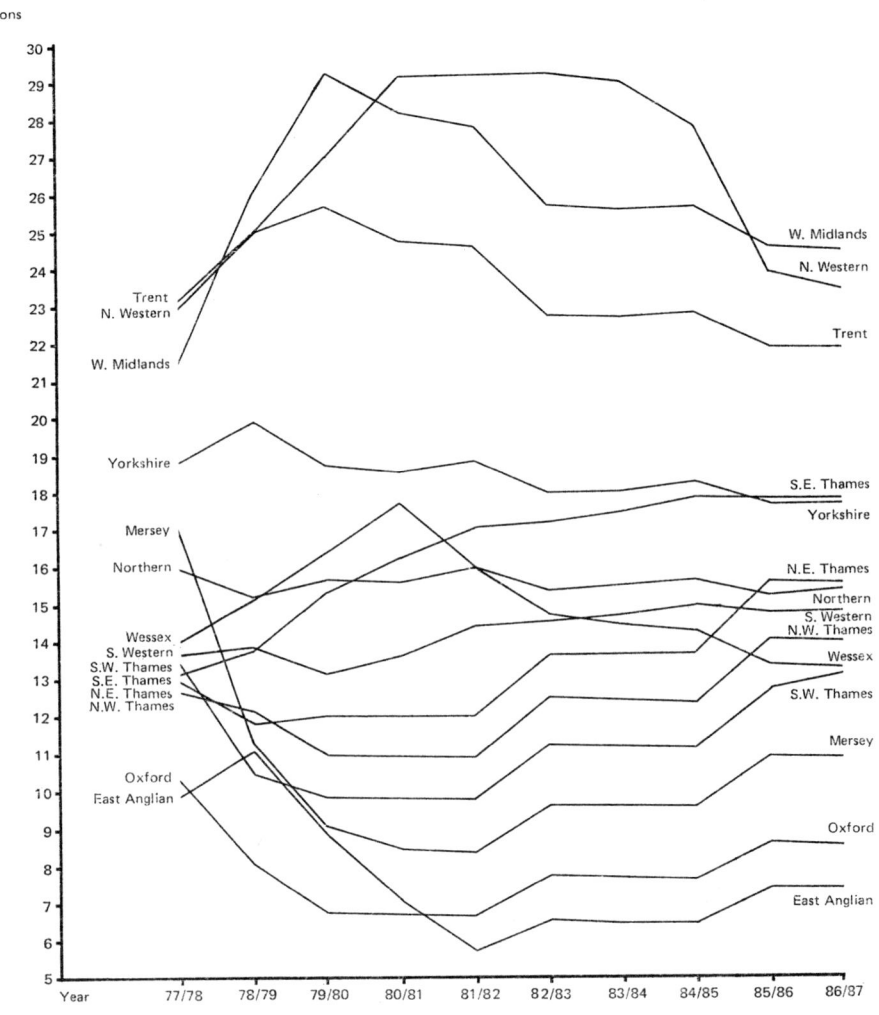

£ millions

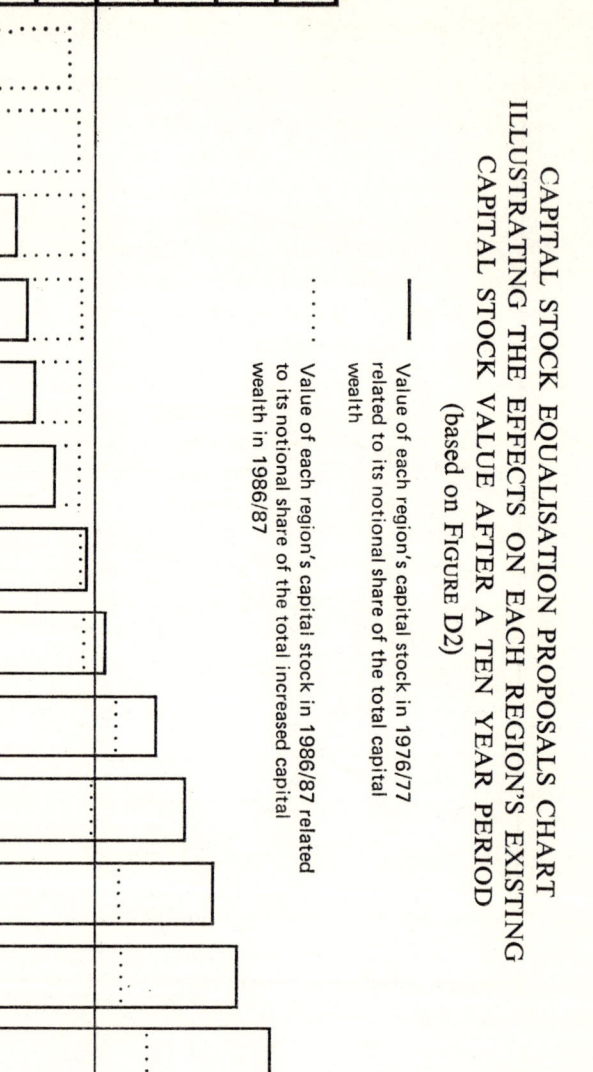

CAPITAL STOCK EQUALISATION PROPOSALS CHART
ILLUSTRATING THE EFFECTS ON EACH REGION'S EXISTING
CAPITAL STOCK VALUE AFTER A TEN YEAR PERIOD
(based on FIGURE D2)

——— Value of each region's capital stock in 1976/77
related to its notional share of the total capital
wealth

········ Value of each region's capital stock in 1986/87
related to its notional share of the total capital
wealth in 1986/87

········ Value of each region's capital stock in 1986/87 related
to its notional share of the total increased capital
wealth in 1986/87

%

120
115
110
105
100 Target
95
90
85

N. Western
Wessex
Trent
W. Midlands
Yorkshire
Northern
S. Western
S.E. Thames
East Anglian
S.W. Thames
Oxford
N.E. Thames
N.W. Thames
Mersey

THE BIDDING APPROACH

E1.   Capital expenditure results in a flow of benefits over the subsequent life of the asset purchased and helps to determine the pattern and quality of services for that period. It is also 'lumpy' in the sense that a major programme represents a substantial proportion of the annual cash flow of a RHA, and even more so for an AHA. There is thus a need for special arrangements to finance the investment. In order to ensure that resources are being rationally used for investment purposes, the flow of expected benefits needs to be related to the once-and-for-all capital outlay. In commercial investment appraisal, known as discounted cash flow, future cash benefits are calculated and discounted at the current rate of interest to give a 'present value'. If this 'present value' exceeds the capital outlay, then the investment is considered to be worthwhile.

E2.   In the health service it is not easy to quantify benefits in terms of cash flows. However it should be possible to consider the relative importance of the benefits from different forms and different levels of capital expenditure and to compare them with the benefits to be derived by providing services by revenue expenditure alone. For example, Authorities could draw up a list of possible capital schemes and rank them in order of priority perhaps for example on the basis of the following categories:

Very urgent
Urgent
Less urgent.

A notional return of, say, 12%, 10% and 8% respectively is applied to each of these categories. This means that for each project marked 'very urgent' the RHA is prepared to sacrifice £134,000 pa out of its revenue for 20 years for each £1m worth of capital. For 'urgent' projects the sacrifice is £117,000 and 'less urgent' £102,000. The total capital sum can then be distributed according to the priorities. Thus those projects rated 'very urgent' are met first. If funds are left, the 'urgent' projects are funded. And 'less urgent' will be considered only if there are any remaining.

E3.   The RHAs with successful bids are committed to making their 'mortgage repayments' in the subsequent years out of their revenue. These repayments are recycled on the basis of the revenue allocation formula. In this way those RHAs which make high bids, that is choose to be capital-intensive, receive the capital at a cost to them of revenue. Other RHAs bid low and so opt for a revenue-intensive service and while they receive less capital they benefit from more revenue in subsequent years.

E4. The main advantages of a bidding approach are considered to be:

E4.1   Authorities are allowed to vary their own ratios of capital/revenue to suit thier preferences, perception of 'need' and the state and condition of thier existing stock.

E4.2   Central decisions do not need to be taken about the relative 'needs' of different RHAs or AHAs.

E4.3   Authorities are encouraged to quantify the benefits of additional capital, as compared with additional revenue expenditure in future years, and this should lead to improved allocation decisions.

E4.4   Under-endowed RHAs can choose to build up the quantity of their stock more rapidly by forgoing part of their revenue allocations. Also RHAs with surplus old stock can borrow capital to provide new facilities of higher quality, close the old hospitals and pay for the capital out of the revenue saved.

E5. Although simple in conception, this approach may be complex to operate, especially in the period of transition towards a more equitable distribution of resources. In particular, as the success of one RHA's bid depends upon the reaction of the other RHAs it would be difficult for Authorities to make long-term plans with certainty. However, this approach has many merits which may make it an attractive proposition in a future period of greater stability, particularly in making allocations to the level of AHAs.

Printed in England for Her Majesty's Stationery Office by Oyez Press Limited
Dd 507290   K200   9/76